O BROTHER

Also by John Niven

O BROTHER

JOHN NIVEN

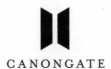

CANONGATE

First published in Great Britain in 2023
by Canongate Books Ltd,
14 High Street, Edinburgh EH1 1TE

canongate.co.uk

1

British Library Cataloguing-in-Publication Data
A catalogue record for this book is available on
request from the British Library

ISBN 978 1 80530 058 8

Typeset in Bembo Std by Palimpsest Book Production Ltd,
Falkirk, Stirlingshire

Printed and bound in Great Britain by Clays Ltd, Elcograf S.p.A.

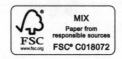

For Robin, Lila, Alexandra and Morty

'For a writer, nothing is ever quite as bad as it is for other people because, however dreadful, it may be of use.'

— Alan Bennett

'Autobiography is only to be trusted when it reveals something disgraceful. A man who gives a good account of himself is probably lying.'

— George Orwell

PART ONE

Tuesday, 31 August 2010

I get the call just after 7am, the call part of me has been expecting for most of my adult life. My then partner Helen is in the kitchen when I walk in, holding our two-year-old daughter Lila with one arm, holding the phone out to me with her free hand. The sage green wallpaper we had in there. The big, stainless-steel fridge freezer behind her. Late-summer sunshine through the windows. 'It's my mum,' she says. 'It's about your brother . . .' I take the phone from her as she watches me in the intense, quizzical way we monitor people who are about to receive Very Bad News. I have learned that we are looking for their reaction, fearful of how it might go. Inwardly I say the words I've had occasion to use many, many times over the years, words my parents had often used too –

Oh, Gary – what have you done now?

'Sheila?'

I am very fond of Helen's mum, who we lived with for nearly four years as I wrote the novels that would become my first two published books. 'John, listen . . .'

Sheila was a doctor, now retired, and while she's upset, a little nervous, she's professional and to the point. She tells me that my mum has just rung her because my mobile has been switched off and she found that the only other number she could remember off by heart was Sheila's landline. My brother is in the intensive care unit at the local hospital, in a coma. My mum is already there. I am to call her right away. She gives me the number for the ICU and I get through to a charge nurse, who tells me that Gary tried to hang himself in the early hours of that morning. He is alive and is being kept in an induced coma for the time being. She cannot find mum but tells me that my younger sister Linda has also been notified and is on her way down to Ayrshire from Glasgow. I remember looking through the glass of the kitchen door, up the length of the garden, to where I had an office at the time, where work was waiting for me, and thinking something like – *finally*. Or – *here it is*.

I book a flight, pack a bag and arrange a hire car. I kiss Helen and Lila goodbye and I get in the cab for the half-hour drive to Heathrow. It is the last day of August and the sky is incredible as I fly through it: an intense cyan blue, what New Yorkers sometimes call '9/11 weather'. I arrive at North Ayrshire District General Hospital, in Crosshouse, just outside Kilmarnock, around 2pm. I have history with this building. It opened in 1984, when I was doing my Highers. My father recovered from his first heart attack here. In my teenage years a friend was hospitalised following a car crash. I have seen aunts and uncles wither and die from cancer in here. It is known to all locals and staff as either simply 'Crosshouse' or 'NADGE'.

And here I was again, coming along a white-walled corridor towards the ICU where my mother and my sister are waiting on chairs. Mum looks desiccated, wrung out, much older than her sixty-seven years, as she collapses into me sobbing. Linda, as is her way, has already

4

established an easy rapport with the nurses. My little sister is thirty-seven, seven years my junior, enough of a gap that we have never had the usual sibling static. We've always been close. She is also, by some margin, the easiest of the three Niven children: warm, outgoing and industrious, happily married and employed and with a small baby girl of her own. I finally get to ask it – 'what happened?'

What happened was this . . .

Gary rang the emergency services in the early hours of that morning, at 4.13am. (Literally the darkest hour before the dawn at that time of year in Scotland.) He said he'd been depressed and had been trying to kill himself. (This account will be corroborated by the transcript of his 999 call, which it will later take me three Freedom of Information requests to obtain.) An ambulance arrived fourteen minutes after his call and the two-man crew spent around a quarter of an hour at his house before he willingly went with them to Crosshouse Hospital – a ten-minute drive from where he lived. I picture him on this journey: conscious, lucid (his arm lacerations were 'superficial'), chatting to the paramedics.

It would have been getting towards 5am as they drove east through the Ayrshire countryside, the Firth of Clyde sparkling somewhere over to their right. The sun would have been coming up in front of them. The day ahead was going to be another beautiful one. Did he notice that? Gary was treated by the charge nurse for the cuts on his arms. He told her about his cluster headaches and how he had been experiencing some severe bouts recently. He needed to breathe oxygen during attacks to abate them. (He'd had a cluster headache in the ambulance on the way to the hospital and had been given oxygen by the crew.) He was triaged as non-urgent and placed in a small room,

5

with the door open for observation, while he waited to see a doctor. At some point he managed to close the door and hang himself using his sweater as a ligature and a doorframe as his makeshift gallows. He hadn't killed himself outright, but his brain had been deprived of oxygen for 'some time' and he had been put into a medically induced coma for the next twenty-four hours, which we learn is standard procedure when dealing with the kind of brain trauma that results from a failed hanging attempt.

A doctor and a member of the hospital administration appear and we are taken to see Gary. And right away I sense a nervousness, a tension fairly crackling off the staff. My brother had, after all, managed to hang himself while in their care. We go into the ICU and there he is: bare-chested, intubated, a ventilator breathing for him, his chest rising and falling in time to the mechanical hum and hiss. A phalanx of monitors surrounds him, with their pale blue twining coils. Always slim, my brother looks painfully thin, his cheeks and temples hollow. He's flushed, with a light sweat on his brow, and he hasn't shaved in a few days. But his face is peaceful, sleeping. The real story unfolds as you look down. There is the red welt of the ligature mark around his neck. The bandages on both forearms, covering the latticework of cuts, cuts we will learn were freshly made that morning. There are also scabs on his bruised knuckles, not unusual for Gary over the years, either from his job as a carpenter, or from the anger that forever seemed to simmer inside him, boiling over onto walls, wardrobes, doors.

I flash on an image of him from seventeen years earlier – Christmas morning, 1993, the first Christmas after dad died – furiously punching the wooden wall of the garage beside my parents' house, the dark, creosoted timber splintering beneath his fists as he wept and raged. We are told about Gary's score on the Glasgow Coma Scale: 3. Not good. It is hoped that the sedative-induced coma will reduce the rate of cerebral blood flow, causing the blood vessels in the brain to narrow, decreasing the space the brain takes up and reducing intracranial pressure, the hope being that the trauma to the brain can be averted, relieved.

Mum looks at the doctor like a child having particle physics explained to them. She pulls her chair up to her son's bedside and settles in for her vigil. Gary is going to come through this. He is going to live and that's that. Incredibly, I fight the urge to laugh. Because I already know about the Glasgow Coma Scale. About comas in general. And the fact that Gary was in a coma in this very hospital seemed to me such a perfect example of life imitating art that it was almost ludicrous.

The year before, in the summer of 2009, I published my third novel, *The Amateurs*, a tale of golf, gangsters and infidelity set in small-town Ayrshire. (It was actually published under the title *Coma* in Germany.) The book revolved around two brothers, Gary and Lee Irvine: Gary was a hopeless amateur golfer and Lee a hopeless amateur gangster. The plot kicker saw Gary – his name a confection of my brother's and the town where we grew up – getting hit on the head with a golf ball and sent into a coma. When he finally wakes up a week later, he discovers that he now has the perfect golf swing, along with other, less desirable and comic side effects: Tourette's Syndrome and chronic priapism. I put the fictional Gary Irvine in a coma in this very hospital and I described the following bedside scene with his mother Cathy . . .

*   *   *

Cathy could only express her feelings in Hallmark-card poetry, in fridge-magnet philosophy, in platitudes and commonplaces; but her feelings were no less real for having been expressed as clichés. The grade, the quality of love she felt for the boy was something the childless, unconscious Gary was still many emotional miles from understanding. As she dabbed with a wet wipe at the dried saliva crusted at the corner of his mouth, his three-day stubble scratching the underside of her wrist, Cathy reflected on how gladly she would have taken his place, for her love for him was fathomless and her will for him to live weighed more than her own soul. So Cathy talked to him, leaving his bedside only to fulfil the bare essentials of her existence: toilet, nicotine, caffeine.

I had written those words three years earlier, in 2007. Now here I was: living it. I was sitting in the very hospital I'd put in the book, watching my mother do all the things for Gary in real life that I'd had Cathy do for the Gary in the book: stroking his hand and whispering softly to him while she watches the monitors as intently as a Wimbledon line umpire stares at their strip of chalk, for any blip or uptick that might represent a stirring, the beginning of Gary simply sitting up and saying 'where am I?'

Or 'what happened?'

Or, more in character, 'WHIT THE FUCK'S THIS PISH? GET IT AFF ME!'

'It can help if you talk to him,' we are told. And mum is already doing this, whispering tearfully to him, asking him about what he's done, why he's done it. Linda and I look at each other, too self-conscious to go there yet.

We will discover that Gary has left no note.

There will be no neat conclusion.

The final page of the book just got ripped out. The last reel burned up. Nabokov said, 'A man who has decided upon self-destruction is far removed from mundane affairs, and to sit down and write his will would be, at that moment, an act just as absurd as winding up one's watch, since together with the man, the whole world is destroyed; the last letter is instantly reduced to dust and, with it, all the postmen.' But, as anyone who has been around it will tell you, the absence of that note pumps more oxygen into the wildfire – the ground zero – of suicide, fuelling its incredibly powerful half-life, its chain reaction of unanswered questions, its unending 'maybes' and 'ifs' and 'should haves'. When a child kills themselves the thought that can break the parent is – where did I go wrong? When the child is one of two or three, that thought often modulates to – why him? Why her? What went so wrong for them?

And these thoughts go on for a lifetime, suicide being, among other things, a Chernobyl of the soul.

These are the thoughts that, more than a decade on, still chase my mother to sleep at night and lie patiently waiting for her in the morning. In the years to come, I find that sometimes, when I watch my own small children – while they play, while they eat – my mind will wander unauthorised and I'll find myself picturing them one day far in the future, long after I am dead, having lost their way, stumbling towards that last outpost, with no hand for them to hold. I see my child (Robin, Lila, Alexandra, even tiny Morty) in the bathtub, testing the edge of the razor blade, wandering by the lonely canal bank, feeling the weight of the damp, mossy stone, stepping up onto that stool, pushing their head through the . . .

You reel back, don't you? If you have children, whenever you get

9

too close to thoughts like these, it feels as though you have sprinted up to a cliff-edge, stopping with your toes dangling over the edge, pebbles scattering down, falling towards the ground thousands of feet below as you totter, windmilling your arms, trying to pull back, your head rushing. My mother's sister, my late Aunt Bell – a family icon, a black belt of the malapropism and the off-kilter phrase – was once told about our younger sister Linda tripping and smashing her milk teeth into fragments on our grandmother's concrete front step. 'Don't!' Bell screamed, stopping up her ears with her fists. 'It makes ma bum go aw fizzy!'

Exactly so, Bell. Your bum fizzes as you shake your head, stop up your ears and blow your cheeks out to chase these thoughts away like a nightmare. And then the rush of relief shooting through you, calming as heroin, as you realise it was just that – just a nightmare – and not reality. As it is for mum, here at the hospital bed, taking Gary's finger-tips in her own.

'Why, son? Why?' mum asks him as she strokes his hand. *'Could ye no talk to me? Ah would have helped ye . . .'*

Linda and I have plenty of questions of our own, and some brewing theories about the 'why?'. But I'm also wondering about the 'how?' And, after what feels like an appropriate amount of time spent respectfully watching the monitors, the drip of the saline, the click and hiss of the respirator, I ask if we can see the room where Gary hung himself. There's a little resistance, some humming and hawing, before Linda and I are taken on a tour of the relevant part of the A&E department. It is shocking to see that the room where it happened is maybe fifteen feet from a nurses' station. We go inside the small room, a cubicle really. It strikes me that it is *festooned* with

10

ligature points. An odd place to leave a patient admitted with suicidal ideation. But then the whole situation is odd: he calls the emergency services because he's suicidal and then suddenly decides to kill himself in the hospital? 'Can we hear his 999 call?' I ask. 'Or see a transcript?'

The administrator goes off, does some conferring and comes back to tell us that the hospital does not have the authority to release that information. Patient confidentiality.

'Actually,' she adds, 'I don't think anyone's ever asked for that before.' I'm unsure whether she is implying I am ghoulish or just pursuing something irrelevant, but it seems a perfectly reasonable question to me. Why wouldn't we want to know everything we could about Gary's state of mind that morning? I make a mental note to find out how you go about getting the transcript of a 999 call. I can see the administrator making her own mental note: *this one's trouble.*

'How long will he stay like this?' I ask the doctor.

'Twenty-four hours. We'll start withdrawing the sedatives tomorrow morning.'

'Then what happens?'

'Well, then we'll see . . .'

Mum behind us – talking to Gary, to dad, to God. Mum, who had just begun to get her life back on track in the last few years, with her new boyfriend Eddie. An 'autumn romance' as they used to call it, fifteen years after dad died.

The coiling lines on the monitors, pale blue – the colour of the foil on the Icebreaker bars dad used to love.

The Questions begin.

How did we get here?

11

As you embark on something like this, as you comb through the years, you are confronted with something like an identity parade of former selves. Here they come, shuffling into the white room, in front of the black horizontal bars, all dressed differently (up until around the age of 40 at any rate), all with slightly different haircuts, different ideas about the world, all awkwardly taking their place in the line-up and squinting at the two-way glass. Aspects of all these personas have been jettisoned along the way to get you to whoever you are now. *The Usual Rejects*. Some of these old versions of you will be more familiar than others, but, for most of us, they will all be shuffling around twitchily to some degree or other. *Guilty*. How do you rate these old selves? Look back ten or fifteen or twenty years. What was that guy like? How would you rank them in the pantheon of former selves? And, as with any decent thriller, it's always the guy you least suspect. In some ways the thirteen-year-old me who joined the Air Training Corps – standing there in uniform, saluting, struggling to shoulder the nine-pound Lee Enfield .303 rifle – is now more recognisable to me than the twenty-seven-year-old waving the champagne bottle above his head as he dances on the balcony of the Chrysler Building, howling at the New York moon, blitzed on cocaine and Quaaludes.

But, still, here they both are, next to each other in the line-up, squinting into the glare, taking their turn stepping forward – '*OK, you deadbeats. Start talking.*'

Some of them you just want to fetch a mug of tea for. To roll out the good cop, the guy who will say, '*Hey, you were young, don't be too hard on yourself kid.*' But there are others, the real offenders, who you want to grab by the lapels and scream, '*Are you kidding me with this shit?*'

You want to reach back through the years and drag them down to the cells, where you will turn off the recording equipment and get busy with the rubber pipe and the rolled telephone book.

Because that's what it feels like to me, the memoir.

A forced confession.

1973

'Too jaggy!'

'Armies uppa sky . . .'

This is the mantra mum uses to get us to put our arms up, so she can slide the vest or sweater down over our heads. (One I still use on my own children, half a lifetime later.) 'Come on, Gary, armies uppa sky.' But he won't. Gary is trying, urgently, to pull away from her as he scrabbles at his feet. 'No . . . no . . . *NO!*' he says. And, with a twist, he is free from her grip and staggering across the room – like a barroom drunk in his tiny vest – as he tears the offending item off.

We are in the bedroom Gary and I share in the flat on Martin Avenue. The orange-and-chocolate carpet. The pine bunk beds with the purple nylon sheets. Two bedrooms, kitchen, living room. Our flat is brand new, built in 1966, the year I was born, and we are its very first occupants. It is on the ground floor, with a tiny square of front garden, and everything about it feels new, modern. It feels like what I didn't know the 60s felt like at the time. But not for much longer: we will leave for a bigger house this summer, when our sister Linda is born.

'Please, son, come on,' mum says as Gary makes a run for it. He trips, going down near the door, Steve McQueen-ing it just at the wire, inches from freedom, and she is upon him, getting him on his back, trying to grab one leg and get the thing back on there. But it's no good, Gary's feet are a blur, his heels frantically thrumming against the carpet, tears springing from his eyes now, screaming like a heretic upon the rack.

'NO! NO! DON'T LIKE IT!'

She catches a leg and manages to begin to get it back on as he scrabbles to get it off again, mum trying to hold him down with her right arm and complete the operation one-handed. I watch, sitting fully dressed on the bottom bunk. Gary is not yet five. I am nearly seven and I am already late for school. In my mind, somewhere down the labyrinth of corridors in the Memory Palace, a song is playing, a song that terrifies me in the early 70s as it talks about how you might wake up in the morning to find that your mama has gone. Jesus Christ. Why would you say that? Why would you even . . . the very *thought* of it. But right now, my mama has warmer matters in hand. Gary is straining and grunting, his back arched like a bow, his heels digging into the carpet, the teeth gritted, the veins in his neck cording, beads of sweat on his forehead. But it's no use. Gary fights the good fight but mum is bigger and stronger and, with a final tug, she manages to pull it back on. It is a brief triumph, however. For she is on her knees and must fumble blindly behind her for his sweater, leaving her with only one hand to restrain the bucking Gary – never more dangerous than when he is cornered in the final stretch. She holds him by the ankle while he twists and writhes like a gaffed marlin. As mum grabs the sweater he kicks out and frees himself again, rolling across the carpet, tearing again at the offending item of clothing as though it were a snake in the process of eating his leg. He rips it off and throws

18

it at mum, who lies opposite him, spent, defeated. Gary pants, sobbing, his face buried in the carpet at my feet. Finally, he swivels around and dramatically levels a trembling finger at the thrown sock – a lawyer identifying the murderer in a courtroom. In a voice ragged from screaming, with a sorrow that is difficult to convey on the page, he says . . . *'too jaggy!'*

'And that was "Chirpy, Chirpy, Cheep, Cheep" by Middle of the Road, here on Radio 1.' Tony Blackburn, the breakfast show. *'It's eight thirty now and time for the news . . .'* Mum gives up and goes off to rescue a dirty but approved pair of non-jaggy socks from the laundry basket.

Later, much later, mum will say that Gary was just like this from a very early age. If the vest or the sock or sweater wasn't just right, he would not bend in wearing it. If he couldn't find a favourite toy, then, rather than play with something else, the toy box would have to be emptied over the floor down to the last Stickle Brick, the whole house turned over in the search operation and Gary becoming increasingly hysterical the whole time.

'He just . . . Gary always wanted what he wanted,' mum says.

The David Copperfield Crap

I was a large, greedy baby, born at 6pm on Sunday, 1 May 1966. 6pm! The cocktail hour! Sunday's child is famously 'bonny and blithe and good and gay.' Of course, additionally, 1 May is May Day, renowned as the beginning of summer in some countries, as a day of festival, rejoicing and celebration in many cultures. It also happened to be my mum's birthday. As her present was handed blinking and mewling to her, Bob Dylan and the Hawks were finishing up their soundcheck in Copenhagen, where they were playing the second date of the European leg of their 'electric' tour. Earlier that afternoon, The Beatles played live in the UK for the last time, at the *NME* Poll Winners' party at Wembley Arena, before returning to Abbey Road, their camaraderie at its high-water mark as they worked on *Revolver*. The England football team were in training for the World Cup they would win later in the summer. The day, the very day of my birth, the cover of *Time* magazine screamed 'LONDON! THE SWINGING CITY!' Obviously, Irvine, Ayrshire, was about as far as you could get from swinging London, but still – good portents abounded.

Gary arrives just over two years later, at 3am on Wednesday, 31 July 1968. 3am, in July: the darkest hour before the dawn. The day he is born The Beatles are in pieces as they record *The White Album*, arguing their way through a fractious overdubbing session for 'Hey Jude', having shut down their ruinous Apple boutique on Baker Street the day before. That evening, *Dad's Army* debuts on British TV. And 1968, Jesus. The Tet Offensive, riots worldwide and the assassinations of King and Kennedy. And Wednesday's child, we are told, is full of woe.

Of course, you can read anything into anything.

And of all these events – all the music and war and death and revolution – the arrival of Captain Mainwaring and co. is the only one likely to have made much impact on my parents' lives down in Irvine.

The Ayrshire town lies on the west coast of Scotland, thirty miles southwest of Glasgow. It has a harbour, a beach and a country park. The oldest buildings in the town centre date back to the sixteenth century. Radiating outwards from the ground zero of the High Street – as if in the concentric circles of a diagram illustrating the blast radius of a nuclear bomb, the kind of diagram that will soon become a feature of our cold war youths – the architecture is Georgian in the first band (the grand old houses along Kilwinning Road that belonged to the merchants) and then Victorian in the second. In the third band, brown pebbledash post-war council houses begin to dominate. In the fourth, as far from ground zero as you can get before you hit the North Ayrshire countryside, there are the newer estates of Castlepark and Bourtreehill, built in the 60s and early 70s, to accommodate the Glasgow overspill, who soon come pouring down. Because, aside from my birth, the other seismic event that befalls Irvine in 1966 is its designation as the last of Scotland's five New Towns. Money begins to flow for infrastructure and housing, and that fourth band rises up to house the people who are fleeing the crumbling tenements of the city for a better life down here on the west coast. There was a real sense amongst original Irvine settlers like my mum that these new big-city interlopers were something to be feared, a threat to their very existence, that a better life for the people from the rough streets of Govan and Ibrox was going to mean a diminishment of theirs. And it *was* a better life down here. The streets of the Castlepark estate – a five-minute walk from our flat – had just been laid, the tiny crystal chips in the black tarmacadam of the pavements like gemstones, the houses themselves white as Polo mints, filled with young families.

Castlepark Primary School opened its doors for the first time in 1970, just a year before I started there. Everything felt like fresh paint and new carpeting. On summer days you'd smell the burnt tar of newly creosoted fences, the sweet, ticklish perfume of cut grass. If you want a visual representation of what a hopeful Scottish New Town looked like in the early 70s, there's no better reference point than Michael Coulter's cinematography on Bill Forsyth's *Gregory's Girl*, filmed in our sister New Town of Cumbernauld. The marmalade dusks filtering through the trees, the colour of the grass and the houses and the bubbling saxophone underpinning everything – they all feel exactly like that time does in my memory.

For we had it good, by 1973. Dad had landed a prestigious job, as site electrician for the building of the new shopping mall in the town, a huge, controversial project that involved the destruction of the old Victorian bridge that spanned the river Irvine and connected the town centre to the railway station and the harbour. The new Rivergate mall would house more than fifty shops and – as a main thoroughfare – be open 24/7, 365 days a year. It was the biggest construction project to ever come to Irvine and proof enough for some that the pendulum had swung too far towards the New Town at the expense of the old. We didn't think that – we thought it was great dad was so involved in something that important.

There was a further surprise when construction was finally finished in late 1975: dad was so familiar with the electrical systems of the 300,000-square-foot unit that the owners, Land Securities, offered him the job of centre manager. It was a huge step up in life for our father: from overalls and crawling under floorboards wiring houses to having his own office, and a secretary, and an assistant manager, and a staff of security guards and cleaners. In the early years the mall was a demanding mistress: the endless call-outs in the middle of the night for triggered alarms, the leaks from flooding in heavy rain, the power cuts and glitches and things forever going on the fritz. Sometimes Gary and I would get to go with dad on one of these, which meant going 'up the spine': the electrical access corridor that ran all the way along the top of the mall, directly above the shopping precinct below, for about a quarter of a mile. It was a tight space, maybe six feet high by four feet wide, and every inch of the walls was packed with wiring, ducts, cables and junction boxes, the weak spotlights of caged bulbs every few yards. A few years later, when I see *Alien* for the first time, the sinister, nightmarish corridors of the *Nostromo* will feel very familiar. It was a source of great pride for us that dad had a job so central to the town. In due course we'd buy our council house, begin to take holidays abroad and a heavy, navy-blue Mark III Cortina would replace dad's old Vauxhall Viva. We were taught to speak 'properly', to say 'house' and not 'hoose'. Our dad, the manager of the mall, didn't go to pubs – to the Turf or the Three Craws – he drank in the bar of the golf club, where he was a member, where he never drank pints, only shorts, whisky and lemonade. Yes, there was definitely the sense, gently inculcated by mum and ludicrous in hindsight, that we were somehow just a cut above our neighbours, above the Glasgow folk.

The Frank and Mia of Livingstone Terrace

Both of our parents were born in Irvine. Dad, John, in 1924 and mum, Jeanette, nearly twenty years later, in 1943. To paraphrase Dylan, right around the time mum was busy being born, dad was busy dying. Or trying very hard to at any rate. He enlisted in the RAF in 1942, at the age of eighteen, desperately wanting to be a pilot. Dad was so keen to fly that he even applied to be a Tail-End Charlie: a rear gunner in a heavy bomber, with a survival rate of something like one in ten by late 1944. These were the guys whose remains were simply hosed out of the glass bubble at the back of the Lancaster, after a Messerschmitt had sneaked up behind them over the Channel.

23

Mercifully, colour-blindness put paid to my father's dream of flying in any capacity and he had to content himself with ground crew, learning his trade as an electrician as he worked his way up to the rank of Leading Aircraftsman, equivalent to a corporal in the army. While still a teenager he saw service in North Africa, Italy and Egypt, although, in childhood, he gave us the impression that his war was largely uneventful. Much later in life, I learned that dad had been engaged during the war to a local girl who was killed in an explosion at Ardeer munitions factory, just along the shore from Irvine harbour. In the way of men of his generation, he never spoke about this. He simply came home in the late 40s and took up a job as an electrician, spending the 50s living what looks to be, from photographs of the period and all available anecdotal evidence, a Sinatraesque bachelordom of golf and Scotch and glamorous holidays.

He is short and stocky, a two-handicap golfer with an infectious, throaty laugh who can turn his hand to any kind of carpentry, electrical or mechanical work. Perhaps more unusually for his time and place, dad is a tactile man. He will hug and kiss us well into our teens and he liked nothing more than a bit of roughhousing on the living-room carpet on a Saturday night, when he came home from the golf. Play-fighting with him on the floor, Gary and I savoured the dad smells: Swarfega and Famous Grouse whisky and Embassy Regal and Old Spice and the faint eraser scent left on his palms by the rubber grips of the clubs.

Mum left school at the age of fifteen and went to work in Boots in Saltcoats, which, to hear her tell it, was the Ayrshire equivalent of Harvey Nichols in the late 50s. Dad was a friend and golfing buddy of her older brother (our uncle, who is, literally, called Bob) and, gradually, during 1964, despite the near twenty-year age gap, their hearts did their thing, and they married in the summer of 1965. The age difference was something we never questioned as children, not even when dad would routinely be referred to as 'your granddad' at parents' night. However, looking at their wedding photographs now, it is impossible to shake the image of the young Elizabeth Taylor staring adoringly at the very-not-young Sid James. You can almost hear dad's cackling laugh coming off the fading black-and-white prints. But it is easy to see what attracted mum: he had travelled the world! He had a car! He took holidays that meant going on an aeroplane! To a twenty-one-year-old Irvine shop girl it must have seemed like Ol' Blue Eyes himself had beamed in direct from the Sands, Sinatra being a cultural lodestone for our parents, as he was for many of their generation. There persists a certain type of Scotsman who insists on 'My Way' being played at their funeral, who views their life as a grand epi-tragic odyssey where they have lived and loved and fought and lost and strived and conquered, while, in reality, having never lived more than five streets from where they were born and drunk in the same pub every weekend for thirty straight years. There's a tendency in the culture towards self-mythology, with lachry-mosity never far behind. (Later in his life, my brother certainly veered into this territory.) And Sinatra would soon eclipse my father in the younger woman stakes, when he marries Mia Farrow, thirty years his junior, in 1966. Unlike Frank and Mia, whose marriage flames out in less than eighteen months, I can unequivocally say that our parents loved each other fiercely for almost thirty years. Routinely – and much to our disgust – we'd find them rolling around like teenagers on the living-room carpet of a Saturday night. A much better time on that carpet, from my and Gary's point of view, was the play-fighting. We'd crawl over dad's mountain range of a body as he pretended to be dead before terrifying us by springing back into life. (Looking back, I'm not sure he was pretending: a phenomenally talented slumber-artist, dad was probably grabbing a swift nap while we clambered over him.) He'd pounce, grabbing us, tickling, his fat fingers (a Z double-plus in ring size I later found out) seeming as thick as our wrists as they dug powerfully, mercilessly, into our thighs and ribcages while we roared with delight. He'd grab both of our faces and hold them close together while he 'beardied' both of us at once, the iron filings of his stubble sand-papering our cheeks, the *Grandstand* theme blaring from the telly behind us, the cartoons over, the sport beginning. We'd marvel at his skin, at the deep, open pores and the seams, like the cracks and crags in a Neolithic rock face. Nearly half a century later I am confronted in the shaving mirror with that same face, that same skin. Whenever a hotel bathroom provides me with one of those hell-mirrors on its expanding metal arm, with its ring of phosphorescent light – more suited to the dentist's surgery or the operating theatre – I am treated to the same view of my own flesh that we must have had of dad's: the nozzles, the manhole covers of the pores, the close-up galaxies of broken blood vessels. The ghost of an electrician, howling in the bones of my face.

The earliest memory I have of Gary and I together is one he would never have: both of us at the window of the flat on Martin Avenue, me standing on the sill, Gary behind me, cradled in dad's arms, who'd got us out of bed at 4am to come and look up at the night sky, where somewhere up above us history was being made: 21 July 1969, Neil Armstrong, taking his first steps from the lunar module, his lead-lined boots *whumfing* into the grey powder.

26

Most of the literature agrees that our earliest memories date from around the age of three and a half. I am three years and three months old. Gary is ten days shy of his first birthday. Of course, the question that attaches itself to all early memories still applies: do I really remember all of this, or has it been implanted by family retelling? Implanted and then burnished and polished up over the years to the point where, half a century later, I can recall it as surely as I can recall this morning's breakfast: the two tiny boys, a toddler and a baby, with their dad behind them, holding the infant, standing close to me, to make sure I do not topple backwards off the ledge. His free arm, the one not cradling Gary, is stretched protectively across my back, to stop me falling off. 'There's men walking around up there,' dad says, pointing to the pewter disc, tapping the window pane. 'Right this minute.' The action is also playing out on the black-and-white TV across the room. And the excitement in dad's voice, completely understandable: his own father, a blacksmith, had been born in 1898, five years before the Wright brothers at Kitty Hawk, when the cobbled streets of Irvine still echoed to the clatter of hooves.

A Friday night in early October 1971. The clocks have not yet gone back, the nights on the west coast of Scotland still light until after nine. Because of this, dad is at the golf course. Me, mum and Gary are in front of the TV at Martin Avenue. Because Friday nights in the autumn of 1971 mean a treat of the highest order . . .

I am five and he is three, and we have our goodies from the ice-cream van — Fry's Turkish Delight, Fry's Peppermint Cream and a whole bottle of Currie's Red Kola — and we are settling down to our new favourite programme. John Barry's stately, graceful theme

27

coils around the opening credits that give us the backstory of the two leads of *The Persuaders*. Lord Brett Sinclair (played with maximum camp by the pre-Bond Roger Moore) is a Harrow and Oxford-educated toff. Danny Wilde (played by Tony Curtis: apparently a true nightmare on the set, he wanted what he wanted) is a tough street kid from the Bronx slums who goes into the oil business via the US Navy. (As you do.) They are both now millionaire playboys and together, naturally, they solve crime. The three of us, on the sofa with the chocolate and the red kola, one on either side of mum, all enthralled at the shots of Monaco and Saint-Tropez and roulette wheels spinning and water skiing and Dom Perignon being poured frothing into stacked towers of champagne coupes and other things that lie far beyond our Ayrshire ken.

Afterwards, in our bedroom with the toy guns, playing Persuaders, I always insist on being Brett Sinclair (likely with a handkerchief knotted around my neck to form a crude cravat), who speaks to the ludicrous pretensions already forming in my tiny mind: that maybe champagne and international travel and roulette aren't completely beyond my grasp. I invariably award the Curtis part to Gary. Soon enough, it starts –

'*Naw, Ah'm no! Shut up! Lee me alane! Ah don't want tae!*'

Mum comes through to break up the squabble.

Gary is always trouble on the set.

How does a sibling dynamic begin to assert itself? How long have you got? How many shelves of books do you want to read on the subject? As first-born children do, I get mum's total, undivided attention for over two years. According to family lore, my first word, at six months, is 'petrol'. I am speaking in complete sentences before my first birthday. I sit on mum's lap in the armchair by the living-room window, Gary gurgling in his cot, as she reads *Harry by the Sea* to me again and again. The perfume of her hair. I can read it on my own by the age of four. Mum gets me a library card, and the first book I choose is about adventures in light aircraft, because I'm going to be in the RAF, like dad was.

Gary is slower to talk – because I do it all for him. Whenever he is asked a question – by a visitor, a friend of my parents, our grandparents – I'll jump in and answer while he's still formulating his response. I speak for him. (*Just like you are now.*) Any question put to the two of us will always be answered first, faster, by me. After a while, Gary just lets this happen. Then, in the summer of 1973, our sister Linda arrives. She's a blonde, angelic baby, the first girl in the family, and strangers will stop mum in the street to coo and gurgle and drop a few coppers into the Silver Cross pram. She also makes Gary the middle child.

And there's another shelf of books for you right there. Middle child theories – it's worth pointing out that they are just that – posit that because the eldest is the most likely to receive privileges and responsibilities, they grow up more confident and assertive. The youngest is pampered and indulged, leaving the middle child with no clear role. They must create one for themselves. Linda can coo and gurgle, I can monologue.

Gary begins to find other ways to take centre stage.

The Power of the Dare

As toddlers our favourite TV programme is *Mary, Mungo and Midge*. The animated series (crude, Soviet propaganda animation) was one of the first attempts by the BBC to reflect 'urban living'. Mary lived on the top floor of a high-rise block in London (a recent rewatch on YouTube reminded me that their flat was south of the river, just on the bank of the Thames around Battersea, making its value today probably into seven figures) with her dog Mungo and her pet mouse, Midge. Each episode featured the trio leaving the apartment to perform some sort of errand. They would descend in the lift and venture out, roaming the London streets without any grown-ups, something that, like 'Chirpy, Chirpy, Cheep, Cheep', always used to fill me with quiet dread. The show only ran for one thirteen-episode season, first broadcast in October 1969, when I was three and a half and Gary fifteen months. A couple of years later, Gary is given a dog on wheels for his birthday: a black-brown beagle, made of rubber foam, with red plastic handlebars protruding from where its floppy ears began and wheels beneath each paw. He is christened 'Mungo' and Gary loves him more than life itself.

Part of Martin Avenue was pedestrianised, with a row of terraced council houses up and down each side and trees spaced along the centre in metal girdles. Pre-school children would play outside all day long in fine weather, mothers watching from the neat front gardens, from behind net curtains or – posher – venetian blinds. The avenue was on a gentle slope that ran from north to south, a gradient of just a few degrees, but enough for Mungo to pick up some speed. While the other children watched, Gary would climb aboard and begin his trundle downhill, pushing with his little feet, gradually going faster and faster, everyone marvelling at his acceleration, at his fearlessness. Then, inevitably, at some point he would lean forward too far, failing to factor in Mungo's already front-heavy design, and there would be the howl as he pitched across the handlebars: the cut lip, the grazed knees, bruised forehead and tears. (As with all small children the wail coming a few seconds after the blood, the astonished intake of breath, the slow ramping up as they take in the magnitude of the injury, of the pain.) And then mum would be there, pulling him to his feet, leading him back towards the flat in disgrace with another lecture on how he was never to do that again. Not least because, at the very bottom of Martin Avenue, lay Patterson Avenue, the sea into which our safe little tributary flowed. And Patterson Avenue was very much not pedestrianised. Here be monsters, the road sharks of the early 70s: Zephyrs and Zodiacs and Allegros and Hunters, in mustards and electric blues and burnt oranges, all snarling and growling past. But, sure enough, the next day, or the day after, Gary would reappear in front of his adoring fans at the crest of Martin Avenue, Mungo squeaking behind him on rubber wheels. Back into the saddle he'd climb, the beast trundling downhill once more, his hangdog, painted-foam face tolerant, forbearing, his eyes expressionless, the other toddlers watching in awe (*'Lookit Gary!'*) but their eyes flickering nervously to those gardens, blinds and curtains, waiting for the parent's call.

'HEY! GARY! GARY NIVEN! NO! STOP! SLOW DOWN!'

Gary – not the type to be stopping or slowing down, rumbling on, faster and faster, the wind blowing through his blond-brown hair, laughing and shrieking.

Wheeeeeee!

We are in the back garden, spinning around in circles. For reasons I cannot, will not, ever be able to remember, we are both holding stones in our fists. Without warning, Gary lets go of one of his stones at the precise moment in his spin that sends it hurtling through the kitchen window, where mum is washing dishes at the sink and gazing out at us. Did it slip from his fingers? Did he throw it deliberately? Can a five-year-old child really understand and be held accountable for their actions? Whatever the reason, I can still hear the glass exploding and the scream that follows.

Thankfully mum is unhurt. Gary will suffer more, later, when dad gets home and utters the words that are already becoming familiar – *'What the hell have you done now?'*

And then the spanking.

Our parents, like many of their generation, did corporal punishment. With dad we'd be thrown across his knee and spanked. On extreme occasions, when she had to take things into her own hands, mum used our spaniel Candy's leash, whipping our legs with the thin, red leather strap. She will often cry during and after she has to discipline us in this way. As we get bigger, and her whippings grow less effective, we'll often have to suppress our laughter as she flails at us.

'Why?' I ask Gary later, both of us sent to bed early after the window smashing, the worst of all punishments, me caught in the crossfire of

Gary's outrage, with the sunshine still coming through the curtains, with the sounds of other children playing outside, the jangle of the ice-cream van, the theme from *The Goodies* and dad's laughter coming up through the floorboards. He just shrugs.

The endless, baking summer of 1976. We're ten and eight now and we are up at Foxes Gate, a pond in the woods on the northern edge of town. Come late spring and early summer it is a hotspot for frog collection by the youth of Irvine, the dark water fairly teeming with them. This particular day, in our efforts to collect as many frogs as possible, we find ourselves foraging alongside a few older kids, including Steven Parker, a boy who lives not far from us. Steven is a few years older than everyone else. This being the 70s we do not yet have terms like 'neurodivergent'. Steven is 'Simple Steven', an older boy happy enough to hang out with smaller children.

Most of us have our shoes and socks off as we wade further into the pond, the concentration of frogs seeming to intensify the further into the water you go. I am up to my thighs when I feel the sensation of something flying over my head, then a splash somewhere ahead of me, and then a cheer going up. I turn to see Gary being lauded by all the others. Indeed, in my memory, he is being lofted up on their shoulders in 'winning the cup final goal scorer' fashion.

He's thrown Steven's shoes into the centre of the pond.

Steven promptly bursts into tears.

We are working-class kids. Shoes are expensive. His mum is going to kill him. Which is why, moments later, I find myself first wading, then swimming, in the cold, murky brown water, trying to recover the shoes.

I am trembling with terror, crying too at this point. If you are aged anywhere between forty-five and sixty, you will know exactly why.

The mid-70s were the Imperial Years of *The Spirit of Dark and Lonely Water*, the terrifying public information film whose appearance on the TV screen would send a generation running screaming from the room. In the ninety-second masterpiece, a hellish, faceless figure (voiced by Donald Pleasence no less, whose soft, ominous phrasing would chill me and Gary all over again a half-decade later in John Carpenter's *Halloween*) in a brown cowl looms in the background, unseen by a laughing group of children playing near water. The voice warns of the dangers of swimming in wild ponds and creeks, of doing, well, exactly what I am doing now. As I swim towards the reeds in the centre of the pond, I am convinced that at any moment I will glimpse the dread figure somewhere on the bank, materialising behind the bigger boys, signalling my doom. I sense my foot snagging on a submerged bedstead, the sudden current taking me under, the bony fingers reaching for my ankle . . .

'The boy is a fool, a show-off. He is trying to find the shoes his little brother threw into the pond because he's a total mentalist . . .'

No, I couldn't quite hear Donald Pleasence saying that.

But I don't drown and, incredibly enough, on my third or fourth dive, I find the shoes. As I emerge from the water, soaked through, I unexpectedly find myself the centre of uproarious cheering. The lads are crowding around me now, reaching out to touch me. Did rescuing Stevie Parker's plastic Timpsons really merit this? It did not.

I am absolutely *covered* in frogs.

It looks like I am wearing some kind of mad frog suit, the sort of battle dress warriors used to fashion from the skin and bones of their enemies. Like the Kurgan, if the Kurgan had been ten and really into frogs. Remembering the feel of the frogs – clinging to my T-shirt, *inside* my T-shirt – and of the glistening tapioca-pudding ropes of their spawn, can still cause me to grit my teeth today. The others fall upon me, stripping me of my luckless amphibian bounty. Luckless because the fate that would befall some of these creatures was often dark. For some of them there would be no gentle, gradual death in a bucket of tap water in the back garden. No, for those taken by the rougher lads – the boys from Winton Road, or the Glasgow overspill boys – their short futures would involve fireworks and cricket bats and tennis rackets: the frog's last view of the world a puzzling, blurring panorama of Ayrshire as it found itself spinning through the blue, having been twanged sixty feet into the air. Death on descent would be instant, however, and preferable to the fate of their fellows who faced the most terrible end of all: slow inflation by rectal straw.

Gary and I begin the long walk home, my feet sopping and squelching as we walk through Eglinton Woods (not knowing that in a few years' time these very woods will offer us greater delights than frogs, when they become the source of many a tattered copy of *Men Only*, *Penthouse* and *Playboy*), past the ruins of the castle and across the poured concrete bridge that takes us over the bypass, the cars fizzing beneath us on the dual carriageway on their way to Ayr, to Glasgow. We come down off the bridge and into Castlepark, a ten- and an eight-year-old boy, their shadows twenty feet long on the baking tarmacadam, the hottest summer in three centuries. My own shoes ruined now, I wonder what I'm going to tell *my* mum. I turn to Gary and once again ask him the traditional question – 'Why?'

Gary shrugs, doesn't look at me. 'They dared me.'

The big boys had dared him. When the devil appeared on one shoulder and the angel on the other, Gary was already fast tending to go with the bolder choice. When the big boys dared me, obviously I didn't dare. Many years later, I will murmur assent when reading an interview with Jarvis Cocker where he talks about his experiences with heroin: 'It's like your mum used to say – "If Martin rolled in dog dirt, would you do it?" Probably. Yeah. If he said it were a good laugh, I would.' Yep. And if so-and-so jumped off a bridge, would you? And, yeah, Gary probably would.

Heroin and big boys making you do it – subjects we'll return to much later, in far grimmer circumstances.

We're standing a few yards behind dad, watching as he settles the club head behind the ball. The third hole at Ravenspark Golf Club was a par five back then, but reachable in two if you hit a good drive, which dad has today. He likes me and Gary to hold his clubs for him between shots as our 'wee hands make the grips sticky', giving him better contact. He's going for it in two, got the 2-iron out. But you know what golfers say – you hold one of them above your head in a lightning storm, because even God can't hit a 2-iron. Dad brings the club down and *punches* it. And it looks good, the ball sailing high, right at the green, two hundred yards away in the purple dusk. But the shot is doomed from the off and dad knows it. It was him who taught us that, when you watch golf on TV, if you can't see where the ball is going, you can tell the quality of the shot from the player's reaction. And now dad's shoulders are slumping as the ball starts to turn to the right, gradually at first, then more severely as the fade becomes a push, then a slice, veering towards the out of bounds on the right. Gary and I tense. Here it comes. *'Jesus fucking Christ, John!'* he screams as he brings the club up like an axe. It's springtime and the Ayrshire turf is still boggy and damp. Dad drives the iron far into the ground, burying it almost up to the grip in what to us is an astonishing show of power. We keep our heads down, like he tells us to do when we, in our turn, are swinging the club. I think today of Gary's scarred knuckles, the fists he drove into walls and doors.

How do you acquire a temper?

You acquire it because someone shows it to you.

Some strings are pulled with the council and, in the summer of 1973, just before Linda is born, we move half a mile towards the town, from band 4 to band 3 of those nuke-blast radii, going from the white new-build flats into one of the brown, post-war pebble-dashes: a semi-detached in the middle of Livingstone Terrace – famous for being the longest street in Irvine. It is the corner plot, with front, back and side gardens and *two* wooden garages to accommodate dad's car and the spoils of his obsessive hoarding.

You come in our new front door and there's a short hallway leading to a small 10x10 kitchen, with a door out onto the back garden. On your right is the door to the living room that runs the length of the house. Opposite the living-room door are the stairs leading up to a small landing with bathroom and two bedrooms off it. The front bedroom, overlooking the street, is large, running the width of the house, and our parents take it. The back bedroom is smaller, and me and Gary's bunks are moved in here along with a cot for baby Linda. Our room overlooks dozens of neighbouring gardens: huts and garages and vegetable patches and toys and tethered dogs here and there.

Dad soon improves this arrangement. He partitions the big front bedroom in half with timber and plasterboard, creating two smaller rooms with a connecting door. One of the new bedrooms is shared by me and Gary, and the other is Linda's. The only downside for Linda is that we must walk through her tiny bedroom to get to ours. But toddlers have little need of privacy so it's not a big problem. And, soon enough, dad improves things even further. He floors the attic and installs an aluminium sliding ladder that comes down from the trapdoor onto the upstairs landing. Our two-bedroom house is now a four-bedroom. The new, windowless attic space (dad is too scared to install a Velux because no planning permission has been obtained for the makeshift conversion) becomes my room for a time, until 1980, when I am too tall, and I move down into Gary's room, Gary taking over the attic space – where he will live on and off until his mid-twenties.

The other big selling point for our parents is that they now have babysitting on tap as we will be living next door to dad's mum and dad, Alec and Lizzie. As a couple our paternal grandparents are a study in contrasts, a Laurel and Hardy deal: papa Niven is tall and thin, nanny Niven, short and stout. Our grandfather the blacksmith is long retired, but Lizzie is a seamstress, who still takes in work, her right foot pumping the wooden board beneath her ancient, manual Singer sewing machine, then, later, the plastic pedal of the electric model dad buys her as a replacement.

They are in their early seventies when we move into the house, but both are still 'good wee drinkers' and will often crack open a half-bottle of Bell's and pour a few stiff ones as they babysit us. Indeed, it is in the act of doing this that nanny Niven first introduces me to the transferred epithet, when she is pouring whisky into one of the 'fancy' Ravenhead glasses dad had got from the petrol station. The glass is dimpled at the bottom, fatter, and she frowns as her pour requires more whisky than she anticipated. 'By God,' she says, 'these are greedy wee glasses!'

As we now live next door, the fence separating the two gardens is removed, creating one large plot. In addition to the two garages there is also our papa's hut, a small pale-blue painted affair with a work-bench, vice and jars of screws and nails, the logos on some of the jars Edwardian, Victorian, having belonged to his father, born in the middle of the nineteenth century. We can come out the front door and roam the front garden before sneaking along between the two garages, around the back of the hut and across the double back gardens. The space seems vast to us, like a country estate. We get our first pet – the pedigree King Charles Spaniel we call 'Candy'. (The dog and our new street forever after providing all the Niven children with a strong showing in any 'work out your porn name' game.) Mum and dad also splash out on a portable TV for their bedroom: an outlandish, unimaginable luxury in the early 70s. It is encased in clean, futuristic white plastic, with the logo *'ULTRA'* embossed in black lettering in the top right-hand corner and it sits on the ottoman at the foot of their bed. As well as two gardens we are now a family with *two* televisions, like something out of the movies. On Saturday mornings, after dad has left for the golf and mum is about the housework, we get to lie in their bed and watch *Glen Michael's Cartoon Cavalcade*, *The Flashing Blade* ('*you've got to fight for what you want, for all that you believe'*) and old Harold Lloyds. When you turn the TV off it takes a while for the screen to die, to crackle away to cold black. Dots and pixels shimmer across it, blips and sparks, like stars dying on the edges of the universe. Under the covers in our bunks, when we are trying to go to sleep at night, Gary and I discover that if you rub your knuckles against your closed eyes, it creates something like the dying of the screen of the portable TV: patterns, starbursts of colour, pulsing violets, nebulae of greens and pale yellows all flicker across the inside of your eyelids. It's like space, like you're pushing through the outer limits of a galaxy, like in *Star Trek*. We call it 'going to Ultra' – interstellar exploration in our own private universe.

One weekend we are playing on their bed, after the cartoons have finished. We're bouncing up and down, gradually getting more and more out of hand. And then the sickening crash, the sound of glass breaking, of tubes smashing. We freeze in terror, crawl to the end of the bed, and stare down . . .

At the ruined portable telly, on its back on the bedroom floor, where it has fallen from the ottoman. Mum runs into the bedroom and gasps, her hand going to her mouth. (My memory wants to add things: wisps of smoke coming from the grilles on the casing of the set.) It is by some distance the worst thing we have ever done and mum barks out the worst of all threats . . .

'*Wait till your father gets home!*'

'No!' I say. 'It wasn't our fault! We–'

It's a situation that will become familiar: me blabbering out the defence while Gary stands mute behind me.

★   ★   ★

Another summer afternoon in the endless summer holidays. We're hanging out in the living room, the blinds drawn against the sun, the windows open to Livingstone Terrace. The lime three-piece suite, the brick fireplace with the mantelpiece, with the inbuilt space for the big (rented) TV, with the little secret compartment that held our insurance policies, our rent book and, later, our passports, the whole thing personally designed and constructed by dad. The heavy dark-wood sideboard with the crystal basket and the big ceramic penguin and the red soda siphon that we never used. It is long into the holiday – August – and we are discovering new depths of being hot, bothered and bored. I am also gradually learning that my little brother's temper – correctly provoked – can lead to hilarious scorched-earth responses. Apropos of nothing I say . . .

'Gary? You know you're a Catholic, don't you?'

'Whit?' A beat. 'Naw, I'm no! Don't talk pish.'

The Protestant/Catholic divide is huge in Ayrshire in the 70s. The first-ever Masonic Lodge in Scotland, the number one Lodge, was established in Kilwinning, just a couple of miles away, where I was born.

Every twelfth of July, Orangemen cram the streets, proclaiming their love of King William and his triumph at the Battle of the Boyne in 1690, all dressed up in their finery. (Look closer and you see the fag burns on the white gloves, the cans protruding from pockets, the stains on the suits.) Back in the 70s the older boys at school echo their fathers with homemade tattoos proclaiming '1690' and 'UDA', King Billy on his white charger crudely inked on forearms.

Our family were notionally Protestants, although this was so laxly enforced as to be almost nonexistent. Dad loved football. He loved watching any sporting contest. (You'd find him glued to the television,

41

transfixed by, say, crown bowling live from Japan.) He could play a bit too. He'd had trials for the local football team Irvine Meadow in his youth. Yet, unusually, he supported no specific side, thus sparing Gary and me the traditional Celtic/Rangers indoctrination. But this way of growing up wasn't without its own problems in Ayrshire. When you were stopped in the street by big boys (as we invariably were at least twice a week during our wanderings in the long summer holidays) the first question you'd be asked was often 'Celtic or Rangers, wee man?' Now, had we been brought up with the normal, useful hatreds we'd have had a fifty-fifty chance in these scenarios. But, as it was, Gary and I would have to reply, truthfully, 'Neither.' So you'd get beaten up anyway. Because you didn't like football and were obviously a 'total bentshot'.

But it was one thing not to be a rabid Rangers fan, something else altogether to actually be a Fenian. Back in the living room I insist to Gary, 'You *are* a Catholic.'

The backstory I furnish him with is long and elaborate, bold enough to make for decent drama yet just grounded enough to be believable. Mum and dad, I tell him, were, of course, Protestants when they married and when I was born. But, shortly after that, when I was just a swaddling baby, a travelling priest came to the door in the dark of night. His powers of persuasion were considerable and he duly converted our gullible parents to the dark art of Catholicism, just before Gary was born. As a result, he was baptised into the hated Church of Rome – a shameful family secret I was finally able to share with him – before mum and dad finally saw the light and converted back to good, honest Protestantism just in time for Linda's birth. 'So, you see, Gary,' I say – doubtless hooking my thumbs into imaginary barrister's robes as I approached the bench for my summing-up – 'you are the only member of the Niven family who was actually born a Roman Catholic.'

Gary goes *bananas.*

He charges out back, where mum and nana are sunbathing, where many of the neighbours are also enjoying the weather in their small squares of garden. Perfectly demented with confusion and rage, Gary literally screams the unlikely question –

'MAW! AM AH A FUCKING PAPE?'

It is the first time one of us has sworn in front of our parents. My mouth is just a tiny 'O' as mum hauls Gary back into the house and does her thing, Candy's red leather leash arcing back and forwards through sunlight made gold-brown by the drawn blinds. Gary's tears and yelps.

Looking back over all of this now, I see that many of Gary's attributes as an adult were in place, in miniature, before he was even ten. Rolling down Martin Avenue on Mungo. Letting go of that stone. Hurling the shoes into the pond. Screaming the f-bomb at mum. The need for attention, the recklessness, the easily-ledness, the urge to prove himself, the fearlessness. They were all there. But they weren't the whole picture.

Graceland, a Film and Two Fights

Dad's brothers were scattered to the winds: Canada and Kilmarnock, Kilmarnock being pretty much as remote as Canada back in the 70s. Mum's siblings lived much closer to home.

Their mother died when they were teenagers – leukaemia – so mum and her sisters were close. She was the youngest of four: Emily and Bell and their brother Bob. In later years, Bob had a tracheotomy, which left him wearing a cravat and removed all the consonants from his voluminous swearing, producing sentences like 'Uck aff ooo uckin unt.' My first wife Stephanie enjoyed this immensely and christened Bob 'Uncle Swearer'. When she was introduced to my great-aunt Eaty – pronounced 'eighty' – Steph misheard this as 'Tay-tay' and assumed it was an Ayrshire variant on 'potato'. For a very long time she thought the name was shorthand for her full handle of Aunt Potato, which, of course, she duly became in family lore. Uncle Swearer and his wife Francis had two boys, our cousins Robert and Brian, a few years older than us, a chasm at that age, and as remote and glamorous as rock stars in their Oxford bags, platforms and furled Bay City Roller haircuts.

Mum's eldest sister, Emily, was married to Uncle John, a man of famously hangdog, indeed Deputy Dawg countenance. Uncle John and Aunt Emily had both worked at 'the Rockware' (a huge glass manufacturer, still there) since the 60s and lived quite close to us in a two-bedroom council house. They never had any children of their own (the reasons never discussed within the family, but, undoubtedly, in a pre-IVF era in a part of the world that tends towards the fates, this was just accepted as another example of 'what wasn't for ye going by ye') and every year, perhaps by way of compensation, they would host drinks and nibbles every Christmas Day.

Aunt Isabel – Bell, the malapropism machine – was the sister immediately above mum in age. Bell found any word beyond the strictly Ayrshire vernacular a near-insurmountable palate challenge. 'Gucci' became 'Goo-shee', 'Sainsbury's' was 'Saints-bury-ees' and, later, the tennis superstar Roger Federer became, variously, 'Feeder-oh', 'Feed-er-ol' or just 'Feed-reerr'. A word like 'paracetamol' could find itself winding up with eight or nine syllables. (While not as preter-naturally gifted as Bell when it comes to hanging, drawing and quartering the English language, my mother can hold her own where foreign words are involved. The simple duo-syllable 'croissant' comes out variously as 'craw-sank', 'crass-ant', or 'crah-sint', the word seeming to have no business being in her mouth and getting spat out as quickly as possible like a bad oyster.) Bell never simply asked to use the bath-room but would inform you that she was 'away for a wee streamy'. By the late 80s Bell and Emily had both filled out a little, their wardrobes a mixture of kaftans, muumuus and crushed velour 'leisure suits': late-period Elvis by way of Monterey Bay maternity wear. It was our cousins on Bell and Drew's side – the Wilsons – who we spent the most time with. The three Wilson children, David, Kevin (I literally had a cousin called Kevin: a high-value pop culture card circa 1980, thanks to The Undertones) and Amanda, were born in the same configuration as us – two boys and then a girl – and we were all around the same age. As kids, David, Gary, Kevin and I were as close as could be, more like four brothers than two sets of cousins. There was a crucial difference though.

The Wilsons were *rich*.

Bell's husband, Uncle Drew, owned a factory, Winton Knitwear, inherited from his father, and by the 70s, he was making garments for retailers like C&A. They lived in a 'bought' house over on the south-eastern side of town, about a five-minute drive but a world away from us. Their place on Whyte Avenue had *four* bedrooms, a vast 30x20 living room festooned with onyx ornamentation, a dark pine sun-lounge extension and a garage that housed a *real pool table*. Mum and Aunt Emily seemed to be forever cooing over some new, high-tech innovation at Whyte Avenue: a deep freeze, a dishwasher, an exercise bike, or a touchtone phone, the smoked grey Trimline that sat in the hall, beamed in from the future. It was very much Graceland to us, a place of unimaginable bounty, with crates of Fresca, Tab and Tennent's in the garage and catering packs of fun-size Bounties and Mars bars in the cupboards, courtesy of the Cash & Carry card that came with the factory. Drew owned a racehorse and a boat, moored over at Troon Marina, and – like that other legendary factory owner of the time, *Coronation Street*'s Mike Baldwin – he drove a fat, sleek Jaguar XJ6 saloon with leather seats, electric windows and an 8-track cartridge player. They took their holidays in exotic locations like Florida, Ibiza and Tenerife. The Wilson house was the locus of many family parties, and Drew and Bell were generous hosts, with trays of food and a Manhattan skyline of spirits bottles.

A typical Saturday night at Whyte Avenue in the summer of 1978: the adults roaring and laughing in the living room, Baccara's 'Yes Sir, I Can Boogie' booming from the house, while, out in the driveway, me, David, Kevin and Gary sit in the Jaguar, playing with the electric windows, the *Grease* soundtrack loud on 8-track cartridge. And here's a guy I'd struggle to pick out of that line-up: the twelve-year-old lustily singing along to 'Greased Lightnin'', joyfully punching extra emphasis into the line about 'tit'. The kid with the side-shed, who thinks he's going to join the RAF and become a pilot, the guy who, after the holidays, will be starting secondary school. Who, in his prepubescent heart, much prefers Sandy *before* her makeover, in her nice cardigan, pleated skirt and pastel-coloured blouses, the Sandy who doesn't smoke. I don't quite recognise that guy. (I'll recognise the guy who replaces him in about a year far, far better.)

Sometimes we'd get to stay over with our cousins and spend the night at Whyte Avenue – always a treat of the very highest magnitude. One New Year, despite offers to the contrary and entreaties not to leave (I remember dad pointing to the lateness of the hour and Uncle Drew, brimming tumbler of iced Bacardi and Tab in hand, responding: *'Time? Time? Do you see any suffering clocks in this house, Jock?'*) we made our way home in a taxi in the early hours, and Gary and I whined at our parents for not letting us stay – 'Why do we have to go home? We *love* staying at their house' – until we finally succeeded in making mum cry. Many years later, watching season five of *The Sopranos*, my cheeks will ignite with shame when Steve Buscemi's character Tony Blundetto is putting his sons to bed in their humble home after a party at Tony and Carmela's mansion and one of his boys says, 'I love where they live. I hate this place.' (The remark has fatal dramatic consequences: it causes Tony B to try to better his financial situation by accepting a contract-killing job for the New York mob, a decision that ultimately crafts his doom at the end of the season.) As I watched the pain falling across Buscemi's face, I sucked air in through my bottom teeth, transported back to that taxi ride across Irvine in the early hours of a January morning in the late 70s, to mum, crying for all she could not give us.

In 1976, *Jaws* mania hits Scotland full force. The film had been released in the USA the previous summer and opened in London six months later, Christmas 1975. Back in those days, however, it seemed to take films an eternity to roll out across the country, and we are into early 1976 when *Jaws* finally comes to Glasgow with its (and this does seem incredible to me today) A rating: equivalent to PG today, meaning children over the age of five are free to see it when accompanied by an adult. Uncle Drew and Aunt Bell take me and my eldest cousin David to see it at the Odeon on Renfield Street. Gary and Kevin, both only eight at the time, are deemed to be still just a bit too young for all of this. I can see us in the stalls now, David and me, leaning forward in the darkness, peering through the skeins of cigarette smoke drifting through the projector beams, as Hooper treads water in the murk, as he shines his torch into that jagged wooden hole. And then the head – the eye dangling by the electrical wiring of the optic nerve. The screams as David and I simultaneously rocket three feet into the air.

Months pass before *Jaws* finally comes to Irvine, to our local cinema, the George. Mum and dad are desperate to see it, and, based on some unknowable, arbitrary factors, a parental decision has been made deeming Gary now *Jaws*-suitable. I, a seasoned pro, will be going to see a film for the second time, the first time I have ever done this. Alec and Lizzie babysit Linda and we head downtown on a Friday night. Only to find that the line is *enormous*, round the block. We take our place and patiently queue, only to be turned away agonisingly close to the front as the cinema is full. The Nivens leave, vowing to return the following night. Saturday rolls around and the four of us head back downtown in the navy Cortina. This time, we gain admission. We load up on treats and take our seats – very near the front – as the lights go down. The black screen. Ominous bubbling. 'A ZANUCK/BROWN PRODUCTION.' I am already aware of butterflies tickling my ribcage, of swallows darting in my stomach. The first two notes of John Williams' dread score rumble up. The camera begins nosing through the weeds and rocks, searching. And . . .

An overwhelming sense of dread floods me. The fact that I have already seen the film is suddenly neither here nor there. I feel hot, panicky. Sick. I am sitting between Gary and dad. I look to my right, to Gary. Of course, he has already noticed, felt, the fear coming off me like radiation. And it is as transmissible as radiation. As we lock eyes, Gary's bottom lip begins to tremble. His hand clutches at mine, which is already gripping the armrest as if on a 747 hurtling down the runway. Onscreen the doomed Chrissie Watkins is running along the beach now, disrobing, soon to dive into the silver water, where, lurking beneath the surface . . . oh, Jesus Christ, its unfathomable size, like a locomotive with butcher knives for teeth. I suddenly know one thing with total certainty: under no circumstances will I survive another viewing of this awful film. I look again at Gary, on the verge of tears now too, and I know that neither will he.

I can get us out of this, wee man.

I turn to dad, my face scrunched up, my breath shallow, tears already springing up as I simply and firmly say four words I should have grown out of – *'I don't like it.'*

'Whit?' dad says through a mouthful of Fry's Chocolate Cream. Mum leans around him and takes one look at the pleading, beseeching faces of her terrified sons.

'You'll have to take them home, John.'

A beat. The tight, controlled venom of dad's *'Right!'*

The word is spat out of the left side of his mouth, through clenched teeth, as he thrusts down his chocolate and leads us to the exit, the sounds of the monster beginning to devour poor Chrissie (poor Susan Backlinie, the actor, strapped into that harness and smashed back and forth in the freezing Atlantic water) hurrying our feet. And then the relief of the bright lights and cool air of the foyer. Dad floors it, burning up Bank Street then Livingstone Terrace on the five-minute drive home. He drops us with our mystified grandparents, and then peels off, roaring back downtown.

Oh, dad. Sitting at my desk today, with Google Maps and the movie playing on my laptop, I can calculate that – with handover time and parking and assuming negligible traffic – you missed roughly fifteen minutes: from the first attack to the town council meeting. You missed the discovery of Chrissie's body – that sickening nest of crabs – and Brody typing 'SHARK ATTACK' in 'Cause of Death'. You missed little Alex Kintner going up like a Roman candle of blood. You missed Spielberg's famous dolly zoom, his homage to *Vertigo*, the seasick lurch the camera makes towards Brody as he watches the horror, as he realises the enormity of the mistake he's

50

made. But you would – *just*, I think – have walked back into the George in time for Quint's arrival. I see you now, coming down the dark aisle, muttering, cursing, searching for your row, apologising as you thread your way through the feet, coats and handbags and sinking gratefully into your seat just as Robert Shaw's nails hit that blackboard. *'You all know me. All know how I earn a living.'* A few years ago, I took your eldest granddaughter to the cinema to see *Jaws*. She was exactly ten too, the same age as I was. You'll be delighted to learn that she coped far better than your son did. Indeed, she was there right to the end, on her feet and cheering when the Chief said, *'Smile, you son of a bitch . . .'* and blew the monster all back to hell. Anyway, wherever you are now on your circuit of eternity, your eldest child apologises for that night. And he thanks you – you showed more forbearance with your children that night than I probably would with mine, with the grandchildren you never met.

Incredibly, even worse awaited me. I strolled into the playground on Monday morning to be hailed by the unforgettable, bellowed greeting:

'NIVEN SHAT HIS PANTS AND GOT TAKEN OOT O' JAWS, MAN!'

And then the gale, the football terrace roar, of the laughter, seemingly the laughter of the entire school. It transpired that many of my fellow Castlepark Primary pupils had been dotted around the cinema on Saturday night and had witnessed our whole, sorry exit. My memory keeps on wanting to add that even the teachers were involved in this mocking. The headmaster, Mr Reid, say, pointing and slapping his thighs with glee as I stood on the asphalt, my face as red as Quint's sun-scorched cheeks, as red as the blood that fountained out of his mouth. At any rate, I would not live this down until secondary school. And, by that point, there would be other stuff to deal with.

As my own children have moved through their schooldays in a middle-class enclave in the southeast of England, I have often found myself struck by how peaceful those days have been. By the sheer absence of physical fights. For you could not credibly get through a working-class childhood in Ayrshire in the 70s without routine violence.

Five rapid to the dome.

Ten of the Na Na.

The dumps.

A boot in the Rab Haws.

Gary and I are digging for worms to go fishing with in the back garden of one of the 'big houses' on Kilwinning Road. Today, these detached Georgian and Victorian villas are among the choicest architecture in Irvine. Back then they seemed to us impossibly grand, so big that you could scale the stone walls at the back of the enormous gardens and steal apples – or dig for worms – with almost no fear of detection. This particular morning another, bigger, boy is doing the same thing nearby. After a while I turn to look in our margarine tub and see that half of our catch of worms is gone. Clearly there can only be one thief. I confront the boy. Who denies it. We shove each other. The rage of injustice boils up inside me and I hit him. We are soon rolling around in the dirt swinging punches until the ruckus summons the owner – the barked 'HEY!' from the distant house – and the three of us are clambering over the wall and running off in different directions.

Gary weeps on the walk home, from the adrenaline, from the trauma of seeing me taking blows on our behalf.

'Ye should just have left it, John!'

I put my arm around him and we walk home along Livingstone Terrace. In the words of Rolf Harris's 'Two Little Boys', the lachrymose tale of brotherly love that was a mega-smash in 1970 when we were both toddlers, *do you think I would leave you crying, when there's room on my horse for two?*

A year later, and the two of us are in Black Mama's, the chip shop, patiently waiting our turn on the brand-new Space Invaders machine. Another boy is playing on it, but we've put our coins in and our credits are sitting there in the bottom right-hand corner of the screen, as the squat monsters advance down in their inexorable left-to-right, right-to-left conga, the bpm of their hellish heart-thump steadily increasing. Gary and I sit talking (what would we have been talking about in 1979? Space Invaders. Or Asteroids. Or Galaxian) as the boy takes longer and longer than expected.

Finally, he relinquishes the controls and begins to saunter out as we eagerly take his place – only to see our credits have vanished. 'Hey!' I say. He turns back and comes straight up to me with a belligerent 'Whit ye saying?'

He's about my age and height, but something in his approach, the glint in his eye, is telling me that he's much more used to violence than I am, that he has seen plenty of it already and is thrilled at the prospect of some more.

'I think, ah, maybe you've taken our credits.'

'Fuck off, ya wee prick.'

There is no attempt at denial. He pushes me.

I push him back.

He punches me in the face. Hard.

Stars, shimmering.

It's immediately clear that this will not be like the other fights, the playground scuffles I have been involved in. It turns out that the rage of injustice will only carry you so far against someone who can *actually fight*. The boy punches me again, in the jaw, then in the stomach, the wind going out of me as I ball into the corner, just trying to cover my face now as the blows keep coming and the yelling and screaming girls come around from behind the fryer, pulling him off me and throwing him out. He loiters outside for a bit, strolling up and down outside the steamed-up window of the fish-and-chip shop, grinning, leering, wanting more, while I dab my face – my swelling lips and bleeding nose – with paper napkins handed to me by the staff. (And it is this, the sympathy of girls not much older than I am, that is almost the most painful part of the whole affair.) And, in the background again – Gary. Crying, trembling, wringing his hands in that way he had when overexcited or distressed. (A mannerism my youngest daughter seems to have inherited. A ghost-genes deal.)

Why am I telling you these stories, this clutch of anecdotes, with their punches and tears, with that small hand reaching for mine in the dark cinema? What are they telling us about my little brother? Yes, he was full of bravado and temper as a child, but he was no nascent Begbie. No instinctive hard case. He wasn't like the kid who pummelled me in the chip shop, the kind of boy who would have happily sat through *Jaws* and far worse. It was definitely there in Gary, early on. I'm not imagining it in hindsight.

The gentleness. The sweetness.

How did it begin to curdle?

If you want to picture a working-class Scottish holiday of the period, imagine the sound of rain drumming on the thin tin roof of a static caravan – forever. The smell of the Calor gas stove, mixing with the sulphur of the match head, just before the *whumf* of lighting. Sometimes with my grandparents in tow, we went on caravan holidays to places like Westward Ho! in Devon, to Silloth in the Lake District and to Anstruther over on the east coast of Scotland. We are in a caravan somewhere like that, me and Gary playing Ludo with nana and papa. Linda, still a toddler, is sleeping in her cot nearby. Mum and dad are out for the night, at the caravan site social club – cabaret, bingo, scampi and chips. Alec and Lizzie have 'taken a drink', as they would have said. An argument starts, something to do with the Ludo, with some rules' violation or a perceived injustice, and Gary is soon at the centre of it, an engine of outrage and grievance. We get sent to bed, our nana (drunkenly, I now realise) tucking us into the single bed we're sharing, still angry about the argument, but mainly with Gary. 'John's a good boy,' she says, patting my cheek. 'But Gary? Gary's a bad wee stick, so he is. *He's a bad wee stick.*'

Many years later, in the aftermath, when the information is of no use to me, I will work my way through a stack of books on child psychology. Some psychologists believe certain 'rebellious personality types' can trace the roots of their behaviour back to a caregiver who would say things like this, criticisms that result in a voice developing within the child's head, one that starts something like – *'you really are a bad wee stick, you know that, right? Why fight it?'* Before our peer group becomes the decisive

55

factor, we base our opinions of ourselves on the opinions of our parents and grandparents. Disappointment from them breeds feelings of rejection and hopelessness: dark, uncomfortable emotions, difficult for anyone to process, let alone kids. So, the child lashes out in anger, with the kinds of behaviour that can eventually untether their lives: self-harm, drugs and alcohol. High-risk activities. The child becomes so consumed by the need to prove the caregiver wrong – or, more destructively, right – that they are compelled to act out aggressively, to mask their deeper pain. These unhealed wounds can fester for a lifetime. Growing up with a negative view of yourself can drive you to try to destroy that self. You tear yourself apart. *'Gary's a bad wee stick.'* Who says this to a seven-year-old? And where was I in all of this? Where was I when my grandmother said these terrible things to Gary? I was right there, lying beside him in bed, listening to nana as Gary just turned away to cry into the wall in his blue nylon pyjamas. The embellishments my mind keeps wanting to add: that I stood up for him. That I protected him, like an older brother should have. That I said 'leave him alone' or 'go away, nana'. But I didn't. I just lay there. I probably thought Gary deserved it. Our family roles were already assigned. I was the 'good boy'. The apple of the eye. Brainy. Studious. Gary was the one who could 'start a fight in an empty house', as dad sometimes said. Not me. Why would I rock the boat?

Saturday night.

Dad is still at the golf club, but will be home soon. Sometimes it's a steak dinner on a Saturday night, with all the trimmings: chips, onion rings, fried mushrooms and the blistered skin of the halved tomato. The steak always well done. But tonight, mum has made her lasagne. The pasta sheets, especially the ones towards the top, are brittle and glassy, splintering apart between your teeth. There will be wine for the grown-ups: the beaming Sisters frolicking against the Alpine blue background of the Blue Nun label. Or the intricate, crenellated patterns – like the fossilised marks of tiny creatures in sea rocks – in the dark brown glass of the hulking bottle of Black Tower, standing menacing and thick-shouldered on the table. Or maybe something impossibly fancy like Hirondelle. (*'An Italian white table wine masquerading under a French name. For supermarket customers it was safe, but with a hint of sophistication. At £1.39 a bottle in 1979, it had the right economic bouquet, though a* Good Food Guide *survey that year rated it as no more than "acceptable".'* – John Cunningham, in *The Guardian*, 2009.) Mum will have dressed up and might be wearing her olive-green catsuit. Music, likely Sinatra, will be playing. My sister – six now – will be toddling around, twirling her majorette baton. Me and Gary will be in front of the TV, where *Grandstand* has finally given way to *Jim'll Fix It*, just before dad gets home.

Mum liked the ceremony of dinner like this, all of us around the dining table at the back of the living room, with the lacy tablecloth, with the 'best' cutlery with the dark wood handles, the 'crystal' glasses, the wine with its paper-napkin cravat. I did too. It all felt impossibly glamorous, until I got to my late teens and started to fancy myself more worldly than my parents, when I began to mock and sneer at their attempts at sophistication.

'You know well-done steak is an abomination, pater?'

I'd have read about it somewhere – in some book – and begun to demand my slice of rump served rare, invariably prompting the response that it would be 'my arse that would be rare' if I didn't shut up and eat what I was given. The seventeen-year-old me: another guy I'd very much like to drag out of that line-up for a few minutes of quality alone time. But that persona is a few years away yet, with his *NME* and his weird music and his books and his arty films.

Later, after *The Generation Game*, Linda is in bed and it's just me and Gary, mum and dad, the four of us having our supper in front of *Kojak*, the last programme we are allowed to watch before bedtime, staying up until nearly eleven o'clock being something of a weekend treat. For us 'supper' meant a plate of buttered toast and a mug of tea last thing at night, a giving-your-kids-caffeine-before-bed scenario that strikes me as utterly insane now. I never heard the word 'supper' in any other context until I moved to London in the early 90s and began to meet middle-class people, when it transpired that supper meant dinner. Although sometimes these folk said 'dinner' too. I once asked an upper-class friend what the exact distinction between 'supper' and 'dinner' was. Supper, she said, tended to be more informal, with fewer people. Dinner was a grander affair. Whatever, I am still unable to say the word 'supper' with a straight face, having long left the working-class Scottish version of tea and toast at bedtime behind and failed to grow into its more aristocratic usage.

The other – far rarer – treat we occasionally had for supper back then was when, after much wheedling, and usually only if he'd had a drink, dad could be prevailed upon to make the only dish he could: potato fritters, or 'scallops'. He'd whip up a huge batch of stiff flour-and-water batter and then dip thick slices of potato in it before dropping them into the frothing mire of the chip pan. (And picture my face, a decade later, in Glasgow's Rogano, when I confronted actual scallops for the first time and found myself looking at two tiny discs of mollusc, rather than the plate of fried potatoes I thought I'd just ordered.) But no potato fritters tonight. We eat our tea and toast and watch Lieutenant Theo Kojak doing his thing on the gritty streets of Manhattan. Telly Savalas mania peaked in the UK around now. You'd see big boys in the town, jutting about, crow-shouldered in their Crombie overcoats, with their gleaming shaved heads. We'd even get a Kojak jigsaw that Christmas: *'Kojak – Crime Story Plus Jigsaw No. 1: The Stinger'*.

I don't know how the argument started that night, watching *Kojak*. Often, with fights and big arguments seen in hindsight, you remember the climax, the peak, vividly. The beginning? Not so much. Because it is often innocuous. A fight about bedtime with an overtired and over-caffeinated child seems the likely cause. But it quickly escalated into a screaming match between Gary and dad, one that ended, as so many did by now, with Gary storming out of the room in a rage. Silence for a bit, the room vibrating with the aftermath, before we hear the cutlery drawer being rattled in the kitchen. Mum, sighing, saying 'Whit the hell is he up tae now?' as she raises herself up from the couch. And then her scream from the hallway. I run out, dad behind me, to see what mum was seeing taking place at the kitchen sink.

Gary – sawing at his left wrist with the breadknife.

Dad's fury is instant and total as he pushes past us, charging in and tearing the (thankfully very blunt) knife out of Gary's grip, Gary kicking and fighting as the flat of dad's right palm smacks him hard, again and again on the backside, on the thighs, on the upper arms. Then Gary, broken, in tears, as mum drags him upstairs to bed, his screams echoing off the Artexed walls of the hallway.

Later, while mum cries in the kitchen, me and dad are in the living room, him trembling with the unspent fight fuel, with the trauma of

59

pummelling his own child. 'That bloody boy,' he says, leaning on the mantelpiece, still getting his breath back, running a hand through his greying hair (he was 55 in 1979, the same age I am as I type this), a catch in his voice. 'Start a fight in an empty house, so he would.' Upstairs, Gary is still weeping and raging. Finally, dad settles back down in front of the television.

And this seems incredible to me now, as I imagine the scenes that would have followed me, or any of my friends, discovering their eleven-year-old attempting to open their veins with a breadknife.

The self-recrimination and the hours of family therapy.

The child psychiatrists and the medication.

Back then? Gary was given a slap on the arse and put to bed.

And, however it gets done, by the time the 70s were ending and the 80s beginning, the family dynamic was well enshrined. I was the 'golden boy'. I studied hard and did well at school. Linda was a 'wee angel', a beaming seven-year-old, with her majorette baton and her cuddles. Gary? 'Start a fight in an empty house, so he would.' Sometimes, once we understand our roles, we seek to expand them.

And the thing is, dad, children are never in empty houses.

PART TWO

Wednesday, 1 September 2010

Another incredible morning: hot and still, the sky blue and cloudless all the way along the west coast, from Ayr to the mouth of the Clyde. We return to the hospital first thing to find that Gary's condition has not changed. There he lies, flushed, surrounded by the sentinels of the machines. His stubble looks a little longer and his ribcage is still rhythmically filling and emptying, rising and falling with the hiss and clank, reminding me of the way he began to puff his chest out as he walked when he was a teenager, the classic pigeon-breasted ned strut, elbows pumping, shoulders jutting, somewhere between a pimp stroll and a power walk, daring the world to get in your way. Mum settles down beside him and starts chattering while Linda and I are taken into an anteroom for another meeting with a member of the administration, this time accompanied by the charge nurse who admitted Gary to A&E the night before. The nurse, who is sweet and nice and clearly still shaken – the fluttering, twitching hands in her lap a pair of shot birds – tells us what we already know in greater detail: that she re-dressed the cuts on his arm, that they really weren't very bad, and then she spent some time talking to him. Gary spoke about not having a job and no prospect of one. About a friend of his who had died recently, in a motorbike accident abroad, and about the increasing severity of his cluster headaches. Calm and conversational throughout, he was consequently 'not deemed a high-risk patient' who required 'one-on-one monitoring'.

I suspect this was a dangerously cavalier diagnosis when it came to a patient admitted primarily because of suicidal ideation. Still, despite having rung 999 because he feared taking his own life, he was not seen by a mental health professional before being left in a small room with the door open, to wait for a doctor to examine him. The charge nurse went off to attend to other patients. Shortly afterwards Gary approached the nurses' station and asked for oxygen to relieve another cluster attack which was looming. He was told he would have to wait until he had been seen by a doctor. He became 'agitated' at this point, saying that the paramedic crew had given him oxygen in the ambulance to help with an attack, so why couldn't they just give it to him now? It was only oxygen. No, he was told, not until the doctor had seen him. Angrily, he gave up and went back into the room. 'At some point' shortly after this, quietly, unobserved, he closed the door. The nurse cannot be precise about how long he had the door shut but that it could only have been 'ten minutes, maybe fifteen max'. Someone eventually noticed the closed door, opened it, and found Gary hanging from the doorframe by his sweater, unconscious and not breathing. They got him down, started CPR immediately, and it took 'approximately' ten minutes for his heartbeat to resume.

'Who was technically responsible for his care when he died?' I ask.

'Well,' the administrator begins, 'we can't answer that properly until we, uh, collate all the statements from the staff who were on duty yesterday.'

Now this – 'collate' – is an enraging piece of bureaucracy that causes my hackles to rise, a term I always associate with *Alien*, with Ash, the murderous 'artificial person' on the *Nostromo*, placed on board by the corporation and played with chilling economy by Ian Holm.

```
            ASH
    I'm still collating.

          RIPLEY
What? You're still 'collating'?
```

'Can we see those statements?'

'Ah, no. But you'll be able to read our report based on the statements.' And obviously, I think but don't say, editorialised. We stand up. 'No one's asked for that before either,' the administrator tells me for the second time in two days. Feeling like a prodigy, I chance my arm with a further question.

'What's the prognosis for Gary now?'

'You'll have to speak to the consultant,' the administrator says. 'He'll be here this afternoon.'

Linda joins mum at the bedside and I go for a walk, trying to clear my head. The forests of signage in a hospital: Admissions, A&E, Cafeteria, Maternity. *Oncology*. What do you have here, in North Ayrshire? Poor people dying, being tended to as well as the NHS can manage. Most of them are inclined to submit to anyone in a position of authority. I think of Gary, deferring meekly to the GP as his cluster headaches were misdiagnosed as migraines for year after year.

I walk outside into the sunshine, even those 'Oncology' signs not deterring me from lighting up. A thousand car windscreens glitter at me in the sun as I pull my phone out and call Helen's brother Fintan, a consultant neuroradiologist at the John Radcliffe Hospital in Oxford. I tell him what has happened and his first questions are: 'How long was his heart stopped for? How long was the brain deprived of oxygen?'

'Somewhere between ten and fifteen minutes.'

The sound of breath being sucked in through bottom teeth. 'Mmm. Not ideal,' he says in the understated way professionals have. 'Have they done CT scans? An MRI?'

'I don't think so. Would you?'

'Definitely.'

'Why?'

'Well, it's hard to say without knowing more, but what your brother's very likely done is effect a massive stroke. I'd want to know how much damage has been done . . .'

There it was for the first time: 'damage'. And the word 'brain' charges towards it in my mind with astonishing speed. This was an outcome no one had articulated yet. That it would not simply be a question of Gary regaining consciousness or not. There was the question of what you might be left with. And this too feels very on-brand. Gary would have to inflict maximum chaos. Total carnage. He was someone who always had difficulty playing by the rules. As they say, any other set of rules might have suited him, but the prevailing ones were no use at all.

I begin to contemplate the possibility that, if he does come out of the coma, there might well be nothing left of the person we know. I go and get Linda and take her out front where we both light up and I bring her up to speed with Fintan's thinking, specifically his reaction to those ten to fifteen minutes when Gary's brain was

66

deprived of oxygen. 'If he does wake up now,' I say, 'it's very possible that he'll have serious brain damage.'

A beat before Linda says, with perfect timing, 'How will we know?' I have never loved my sister more than at that moment. We both crack up. Then she sighs, *'Oh, Gary,'* and cries quietly. After a moment, she turns to the practical, already two moves ahead of me. 'We need to get up to his house.'

'Eh? What for?'

'Uh, John, there might be stuff we need to, like, move?'

We tell mum that Gary might need some fresh clothes, for when he comes round, a fiction she eagerly believes, and she gives us her key to his place. We leave her to her vigil, get in the hire car and drive the ten minutes to Bourtreehill on the northeastern edge of Irvine, retracing the route that Gary would have travelled in the ambulance the day before. It's an area I know from my youth: I was briefly a milk boy at the age of fifteen and I used to make deliveries here, saving up the money to buy my first electric guitar.

This would have been the *Gregory's Girl* period, when the estate was brand new, was still in fact being built. Thirty years later, it is now the third generation of families to live here and the Bill Forsyth bloom is long off the rose. The fresh white houses are now streaked a dirty brown and many of the gardens are overgrown with weeds, their fences smashed. The first thing we see as we come up the path confirms Linda's intuition that a visit was a good idea. There is yellow 'STRATHCLYDE POLICE' tape across the front door and the door itself is blackened with kick marks. We look at each other. The door is closed and locked. But the key works. We pull the tape aside and go in.

It strikes you immediately that the house is cool, cold even, despite the warm, late-summer day. The short hallway has a staircase on our left, a door to the kitchen on our right and the living room, where we are headed, straight ahead. The floor is laminate wood, laid by Gary himself. Two black pleather sofas sit in an 'L' shape around the focal point of the room: the big TV, with the Xbox below it. There's a dark glass coffee table. On the wall above the TV is a movie poster, in a cheap black plastic frame of an icon much beloved by the provincial drug dealer: Al Pacino as Tony Montana in *Scarface*, numb with cocaine, slumped at his desk. In the corner sits a black metal tank – like you would see strapped to a scuba diver. The oxygen Gary needs to abate his cluster headaches. On closer inspection we discover that it is empty and has probably been empty for some time: the task of managing his medication, of lugging the tank to the pharmacy on the bus, to have it refilled, increasingly beyond him. In the unit below the TV is a small stack of books: *How to Grow Cannabis*, *Mr Nice* by Howard Marks, Andy McNab's *Bravo Two Zero* and the three novels I have published at that point. On the same shelf sit two photographs in wooden frames: my children. My daughter Lila as a baby, taken the previous summer, and my son Robin, aged thirteen, grinning, strumming a Fender Telecaster. I remembered sending them to Gary only a year or so ago, enclosing them along with a cheque. He hadn't seen Robin in a long time and had never met Lila. He hadn't thanked me for the cheque or commented on the photographs and I'd wondered at the time if he'd ever got the letter. I pick one of the frames up and, as I finger it, I realise from its rough wooden edges and unfinished feel that it is homemade . . .

I find I need to sit down heavily on the sofa as the thought of Gary making these frames with his own hands breaks over me. The carpentry, the work he could no longer be paid to do, going into this.

'Oh Jesus, Gary,' Linda sighs from the dining table. I go over and see the drift of brown mail, letters in red ink spilling from gutted manila envelopes . . .

'FINAL DEMAND'

'IF YOU ARE UNABLE TO PAY . . .'

'IT IS IMPORTANT YOU CONTACT US URGENTLY . . .'

'OUR DEBT COLLECTION AGENCY WILL . . .'

Credit cards, loans, mortgage, gas and electricity.

The headaches, that police tape.

Everything was falling in on him.

The unpaid electricity bill reminds me of how cold the house is. The actual walls themselves are cold. Linda tries a light switch and gets nothing. We go to the fuse box and try to turn the power on but cannot. It has a purple key thing that you have to top up at a local shop (power by pay-as-you-go, which I will learn later is the most expensive way possible to pay for electricity, a horror-tax on the poor) and it seems that Gary is out of credit. How long has this been the case? Was he sitting in here in the dark in the evenings, unable to watch TV or play his Xbox? Unable to even read a book except by candlelight? Unable to cook a meal?

We sift through the mail, through the debts. Most of the figures involved are in the hundreds of pounds. A few, one of the credit cards, a loan, are in the low thousands. As we tot them up, the realisation dawns on me that Gary has hanged himself (in part) because of a sum just into five figures. It is this that causes me to slide down the wall as I finally start to cry – '*you stupid wee bastard, you stupid wee bastard*'.

The guilt is sharp and immediate, and something about its incredible power is ominous. It is as though it is saying – '*Get used to this, pal. I am going to be around for a very, very long time . . .*' Because forget the few hundred here and there I lent him (grudgingly, always with a lecture), I could have written a cheque to cover all of this.

Linda is crying now too as she organises the bills, stacking them in piles, the born administrator trying to impose some sort of order on a life in freefall. I find myself staring at the drift of hell on the table, wondering how often something very like it features in the tableaux of suicide. Is it generic? A cliché?

O brother – was it just about the money? Come back. Give me five minutes. We can work something out. This can't be it. There were things I needed to say.

We continue our search, deciding to check the garage next. We go out into the front garden, swing the metal door up, and it's my turn to say, 'Oh Jesus.'

It is empty (Gary had no car, never passed his test) save for a few tools scattered around. There, in the middle of the breeze-blocked space, stands a metal stepladder and, dangling from a metal cross-beam in the roof, a noose, fashioned from a thin, blue nylon clothesline. Had Gary tied it shortly before he called 999 yesterday morning? Had he had it up for a while? As a sort of stand-by mechanism? A last-resort failsafe solution? Why not use this set-up rather than something as makeshift as his own sweater in a room off A&E? It would surely have been more efficient. Certainly, more private. Was he going to use this noose and then something changed his mind? Did he realise he wanted to live and then he called the ambulance? Had he decided he just couldn't cope another day and hospital was the best place for him? I add all of these to a list in my head, a list that will come to be called 'The Questions That Will Never Be Answered'.

I climb the metal ladder towards the noose – conscious of the fact I am following in my little brother's footsteps when he ascended to put it up – and try to untie the knot before giving up and cutting it with the knife Linda brings from the kitchen, both of us crying again as we think about the same things. About how it must have been going for him recently in this house. Hungry. Cold. Tired. Penniless. Plagued with headaches. With fresh hell landing softly on the doormat every morning, the clack of the letterbox your personal chimes of doom.

We head back inside and go upstairs.

Everything is neat and orderly. The towels are folded in the bathroom. Piles of laundry sit on the bed in the guest bedroom. In Gary's room, his bed is made and his slippers lie snug by the side, awaiting his feet. On a hunch I get down and look underneath. There, glinting in the dust and dark, is a huge samurai sword, of the kind Bruce Willis's Butch chose when he went back to rescue Marsellus Wallace, a reference point Gary would have appreciated. I am wondering about why he might have felt the need to have this thing so close to hand when, from the other side of the room, Linda lets out a short scream. A mouse, I think, as I stand up to see that she's opened the drawer of his bedside cabinet and recoiled as if it contained a live serpent. I walk around the bed and look inside.

Sitting in the drawer is a chrome handgun.

1978

Herb Albert's Tijuana Beatles

With over a thousand pupils, Ravenspark Academy really is 'the big school'. It opened in 1969, becoming Irvine's second secondary, after the (posher, Victorian) Irvine Royal Academy just along the road. It was built to help accommodate the Glasgow overspill and it is *huge*. Playground legend has it that (like Kelvingrove Art Gallery in Glasgow) Ravenspark was built back to front. Because the main five-storey block of the school which houses everything from the library to the English, History, Maths, and Languages classrooms – academic subjects you might want some quiet for – faces Kilwinning Road, the main drag into town, with constant, thundering traffic. Meanwhile the single-storey complex at the rear, overlooking the quiet of the playing fields, has the metalwork, woodwork, art and home economics classrooms: the 'doughball' subjects, where traffic noise would be less of a problem. Again, like Kelvingrove, the architect was said to have killed himself by leaping from the roof when he saw what had been done to his vision. Naturally – like the Kelvingrove story – this all turns out to be a pack of utter nonsense. However, I soon understand the architect's suicidal impulse.

Because I am *terrified* at Ravenspark.

I am a small boy still many miles from puberty who is suddenly thrust into a world where six-foot fifteen-year-olds who could comfortably pass for Tom Selleck stride about unchecked. A further problem is that I have no tribe. In August 1978 when I walked through the gates for the first time, you were either a ned (fighting and chart music), a punk (the fag end of punk, the Sham 69/UK Subs/Angelic Upstarts end) or a mod (thinner on the ground that summer than they will be the following year, when *Quadrophenia* is released). And here was me: alarmingly, terrifyingly conventional, with my side-shed, my blazer (or barathea, as everyone seemed to call it at the big school), my RAF obsession and my golf. Like a youthful Alan Partridge, I *liked* wearing a tie to school. And, unthinkably, I liked books. When I am eleven or twelve, the first things I begin to read outside the school curriculum are novelisations of movies: *Star Wars* and then *Alien* (which I read long before I see the film), both written by Alan Dean Foster, who will go on to become a fantasy and sci-fi superstar in his own right. Thinking it to be a straight-up retelling of the film, I read Peter Benchley's *Jaws* and am shattered – heartbroken – when Hooper is revealed to be having an affair with Brody's wife. (The first sex scenes I ever read, making me all queasy and fevered.) I'm further destroyed at the end of the book when Hooper dies, the shark's butcher-knife teeth just reaching him in that underwater cage. Spielberg obviously lost all of this in the movie, charitably attributing the whole Ellen Brody/Hooper affair subplot to 'bad editorial advice'. (Others have more bluntly attributed its failure to 'bad writing'.) But I don't know any of this. I even read Hank Searls' novelisation of *Jaws 2*, after dad takes us all to the George again to see it. (No tearful exits are involved in this viewing, with me and Gary there right to the end, cheering

76

with joy when the shark crunches down on that electrical cable.) While I'm kind of aware that none of this is exactly literature, somehow or other it starts to happen – by my teens I am making the weekly trip to the library with mum and am never without a book. Which attracts the kind of random violence Ravenspark Academy does so well. Walking down the corridor, it is by no means an unusual occurrence for one of the Tom Sellecks to just lash out and give you a dead arm. Or a dead leg – viciously driving a kneecap into the fleshy centre of your thigh. Another favourite is to simply hawk a mouthful of spit into your face as you pass by, with much kudos awarded for the last-minute casualness with which this is done: breaking conversation with their pal just as they pass to launch a 'massive grogger' right into your 'coupon'. The first time this happens to me, when Big Rab spits in my face as he passes, I simply stop in my tracks, stunned, saliva dripping from my nose and chin.

As I was increasingly saying to Gary – why?

Part of the reason I have no tribe is because pop music has yet to establish any sort of foothold in my life. Our parents don't really do the stuff at all. Dad was already in his forties when I was born. He'd come of age in the services in the 40s, with Glen Miller and The Andrews Sisters. He'd already turned thirty when Elvis arrived, missing rock and roll entirely.

Mum was still, just, a teenager when 'Please Please Me' was released in January 1963 and Beatlemania began to sweep through the UK, so you'd have thought was much better placed to jump in with both feet. But no. She managed to resist the charms of Lennon and McCartney's work entirely until August 1966, when she finally caved and bought the only Beatles record that we would ever own: a 7-inch of 'Yellow Submarine', purchased for the three-month-old me. If pushed, she'd tell you she 'quite liked' Paul.

And that really was about the penetration of the swinging sixties around our way. Dad did own a stereo, however, with a powerful old valve amplifier – the coppery smell of grilling toast when it warmed up – and a handful of vinyl albums, so bizarrely curated as to almost constitute some sort of art experiment. Aside from their beloved Sinatra, there was Acker Bilk's *Strangers On The Shore*, often played at the weekend and responsible for the fact that the mournful sound of the clarinet can still transport me to Sunday-evening levels of boredom and depression today. There was the soundtrack of *Hair*, the 1968 Broadway musical sensation featuring naked hippies, the ubiquity of its lead track 'The Age Of Aquarius' likely motivating the purchase. And then there was Herb Albert and his Tijuana Brass. You laugh out there – the dear, the gentle – but I'd remind you that in the late 60s Herb was outselling The Beatles (who, as you'll remember, he covered heavily) by a margin of two to one. Now there's your silent majority. Herb is an artist my father will love unconditionally for the rest of his life: by 1984, by the time I have passed my test and am regularly borrowing the car (the silver Vauxhall Nova that replaces the Cortina) I will automatically eject a Herb Albert cassette whenever I get behind the wheel, replacing it with a C90 with felt-tipped title on the label: *Heaven Up Here, Power, Corruption And Lies, The Smiths, Rattlesnakes*.

But before all this, our personal favourite is Geoff Love and His Orchestra's *Big War Movie Themes*. Now, for me and Gary, this was the real Saturday morning stuff, proper running-around-the-house-with-your-arms-outstretched-pretending-to-be-a-De-Havilland-Mosquito music.

('633 Squadron' being, as any serious aficionado of the genre will tell you, handily superior to the more-lauded 'Dam Busters' theme.) As the 70s unfolded, mum would occasionally bring home a 7-inch single from town on a Saturday, usually whatever happened to be number one that week: 'Under The Moon Of Love' by creaking Teds Showaddywaddy, 'Mull Of Kintyre' by that Paul she quite liked, or cherubic Mormon Little Jimmy Osmond squeaking 'Long Haired Lover From Liverpool'. When it came to the canon, mum continued the trend she'd begun with 'Yellow Submarine', where towering legacy artists were represented purely by their novelty records.

Johnny Cash – 'A Boy Named Sue'.
Chuck Berry – 'My Ding-A-Ling'.
David Bowie – 'The Laughing Gnome'.
God, did I need an older brother.

It's tempting to say that, in other teenage matters, I was as much of a late developer as I was with music. But an audit of the facts doesn't bear this out. Because today, with the help of the Internet, I can date the moment precisely.

In the autumn of 1976 Gary, dad and I become obsessed with a new TV programme. Every Sunday night, there we are: dad in his armchair, us sprawled on the living-room carpet, the three of us glued to the screen as Laurie Johnson's music blares out, the stirring brass and trammelling military snare announcing the beginning of *The New Avengers*. Now Gary is a straight-up Gambit man: tough, unpredictable, rogue. Something of the gypsy about him. As with Lord Brett Sinclair in *The Persuaders* five years earlier, Steed obviously speaks to my toff/

officer–class pretensions. Purdey, played by Joanna Lumley, doesn't really factor into our thinking much.

At first.

Then along comes the sixth show of season one, 'Target!', which takes place on a training range, a warren of derelict buildings where agents engage in gunfights with robotic, Westworld-style enemies. Purdey finds herself faced with a steep climb up a drainpipe. The camera holds in a tight close-up on her brown leather cowboy boots. And then pulls back to reveal they are in fact empty. We pan up to show Purdey is shimmying up that drainpipe, having kicked her boots off to assist her ascent. It's not all the shot gives us: we are allowed a good three seconds of Lumley's brown thighs, encased in white silk stockings. Without warning I find myself squirming into the carpet, a bit feverish, with something that feels like a billion tiny fireflies sparkling in my chest. And a less fecund feeling going on further down: something like molten lead abruptly being pumped into what mum calls 'my winkie'. Now, IMDb informs me that 'Target!' was first broadcast on UK television on Sunday, 7 November 1976, five months before my eleventh birthday: clear proof that I wasn't quite as slow to develop in this area as I imagined.

It is the first sighting of the good ship Onanism, and, frothing behind her like refuse following a trawler, the hellish wake of soiled bog roll, tissues and cracked socks. The navy-blue Scotland 1978 World Cup top with the diamond patterns down the sleeves that will eventually become batik. And all the other stuff I didn't know about that was going on around the world on the night of 7 November 1976, stuff that would also end up changing the course of my life. Down in London, off Marble Arch, three young men whose music will end up being kind of responsible for everything that happens to me next, were in a recording studio together for the very first time, finishing up their first attempt at a song that, three years from now, will stop dad horrified in his tracks and cause him to sarcastically do an impression of a crying baby along to the chorus – *WAH! WAH! WAH WAH!* This, oddly enough, will also be the critic Jon Savage's initial impression, when he hears the song for the first time.

Get Some In

The school dining hall at lunchtime is especially terrifying: a scrum of peer groups and noise and jostling and dear-God-where-do-you-sit? I decline the option of school meals and make the fifteen-minute walk home, which gives me exactly thirty minutes to have lunch with mum: tinned Heinz spaghetti or ravioli (best of all: meatballs. Worst: macaroni) on toast. The meal will be eaten on our laps while we watch *Pebble Mill at One.*

Gary fares much better when he arrives at Ravenspark a couple of years later. He immediately elects to have school dinners for one thing, having no problem finding his place at those deafening tables. He plays football and makes the team. He is less concerned with parent-pleasing, more concerned with· pleasing himself, or his peer group at any rate. Where a bad report card will send me into a fug of guilt and self-recrimination, Gary doesn't really care. Gary is 'gallus'. (Scots colloquial: *bold, cheeky or flashy.*) In many ways, although he is not yet a teenager, Gary already has more of the attributes of one than I do. And then there's his features – sharper, more angular than mine. I am still lumbered with a ball-faced blob of puppy fat. Like the childish signature I

81

think will one day magically transform itself into perfect copperplate script, I don't yet know I will be forever lumbered with it. Obviously, all of this conspires to make Gary way, way cooler and more popular than me. Yes, I am definitely troubled by the feeling that I might very much be Potsie to his Fonz.

As if to ram home this point, as soon as I turn thirteen, in May 1979, I join the Irvine branch of the ATC: the Air Training Corps. It is, I reason, bound to look good a few years from now on my RAF application. Bound to help me in becoming a pilot. An officer and a gentleman. I pledge allegiance to Queen and Country and, twice a week, I go to the drill hall on East Road in my blues, with my beret and polished black shoes, and march around, being shouted at by officers and the older cadets. Among the latter group is a guy with thick, curly black hair, olive skin and dark brown eyes. Sergeant Pieroni is seventeen and, in common with the rest of the NCO cadets, he is *mean*. Like the trustees culled from the prisoners in the gulag, these lads are often crueller to us, their own kind, than the officers are. We are schooled in the harsh mundanity of military life: scrubbing floors, learning drills, marching with the massive (deactivated) Lee Enfield rifles, the brass cartridges as big as your index finger, the guns hold-overs from World War Two, from my father's time. But there's fun stuff too: we get to shoot on the range with ancient Martini action .22 rifles, the kind of weapons last used in the Boer War. The sharp, match-head smell of the burnt cordite, the cold, concrete floor on your tummy. And, of course, all of this – the school tie, the golf, the ATC – is intended to please an audience of one.

Dad! Look how much I'm like you!

All around me at school there are the parkas with RAF roundels on the back (a blasphemy I disapproved of), or the black PVC bomber jackets with badges bearing the names of strange-sounding bands: The Skids, The Police, The Vibrators, 999. Armbands that had the letter 'A' in white on a black background, with a circle around it. Trousers with strange straps connecting to the legs by 'D' rings. At the end of 1978, while many of my classmates are getting to grips with, say, *All Mod Cons*, *New Boots And Panties!!* and *Parallel Lines*, the albums the Niven children receive for Christmas are *Father Abraham In Smurfland* and Boney M.'s *Nightflight To Venus*. Apart from mum's mystifying, haphazard 7-inch purchases there will be no other input. Until the following autumn when, early in the first term of my second year at Ravenspark, a boy called Craig Russell sits next to me in German.

Now, I'd taken German because I'd obviously be needing it when I was stationed there as an RAF pilot. As 1978 turned into 1979 I'd noticed that Craig Russell, like a few of the other boys – Keith Martin and Allan Carruthers, both of whom I knew from primary school – had started getting 'a bit punky'. Nothing outrageous – no bumflaps or bondage trousers yet – just an increasing number of badges on their red-tartan-checked lumber jackets or their black Harringtons. One of the badges on Craig's grey leather bomber jacket said 'The Sex Pistols'. Now, I'd heard of the Sex Pistols. They'd been in the *Daily Record*, my parents' favoured tabloid. And they were bad. 'Absolutely disgusting', according to mum. 'That's no music,' dad said. I knew that one of the Sex Pistols had died at the beginning of the year, the guy whose name you saw on lots of the badges, standing bow-legged in a white jacket and aiming a gun. Big Rab – the face-spitter – was a punk too now and he had even written a poem commemorating the death of this man in English class and it had gone up on the wall, presumably because it likely constituted the only piece of creative work Rab had ever delivered on. The words had been written to fit into the shape of a crude coffin he'd drawn, and I can recite them to this day. Admittedly this is no great feat as Rab's 'SID' was hardly 'The Rape of the Lock' . . .

Sid is dead
But not for me
Because I know
Sid did it his way

There is some poetry here, in the starkness of the blank verse, in the teasing assonance of 'me' and 'way'. It might not be Pope, but with hindsight Rab was possibly a closeted e. e. cummings fan. The last line was a reference to the Sid Vicious version of the Sinatra standard, another piece of music that would soon be causing dad to drop the newspaper in sheer disbelief when I played it on our living-room stereo. But this was all to come. For I had never yet bought a record myself. For that to happen Craig would first have to turn to me in Mr McCreath's German class and utter the magic words: 'Hey, Niven. Do you want to come back to my bit after school and listen to some records?'

Which he duly says in September 1979.

Craig is part of mum's dreaded Glasgow overspill and he lives in Castlepark. Unusually for the time and place, his parents are divorced and, even more unusually, he lives not with his mother but with his father and his older brother Steven. Puzzled about this strange invite to go and listen to records, but very much on the lookout for any kind of friendship at this point, I accept.

Walking into their house I am immediately struck by the differences from our own home. There is the strange smell of something like warm turpentine, from the paraffin heaters scattered throughout, like squat, brown weird-smelling robots. In the living room they have an incredibly modern Amstrad music centre, with twin cassette player, record deck and radio, all sleek and silver-faced, magically soft-ejecting and combined in one fake wood unit. They even have a SodaStream in the kitchen, an item as exotic and aspirational to me in 1979 as a sauna, a sunken living room, a walk-in humidor, a private jet. I watch, fascinated, as Craig makes us a couple of bottles of lemonade before we head up to his room. Coming along the upstairs hallway there's another strange smell, a sweetish, sickly perfume coming out of his big brother's room, what I will later learn are the scents of joss sticks and patchouli oil. I glance inside the open door: every inch of wall space is *covered* in posters. There are strange rune symbols – 'ZOFO' – and a disturbing one of a man dressed in schoolboy's uniform, sticking a guitar into his stomach, with blood coming out. It scares me. At the end of the hallway Craig opens the door to his own bedroom and I am astonished to see that his walls are completely covered in posters too. A huge, glossy colour landscape 60x30 of two men with guitars dominates, looking down over the record player. (His own record player! In his room!) The men are both sweating heavily under multi-coloured stagelights and one of them – the one singing at the microphone as well as playing a battered black guitar – has a white shirt on with a blue-and-yellow radiation symbol painted on it. A silver sticker on his guitar bears the strange phrase 'IGNORE

85

ALIEN ORDERS'. And, lined up beside the record player are *tons* of records. All bearing the names of bands I've previously only seen on badges and jotters at school: Spizzenergi, The Angelic Upstarts, The Cockney Rejects. For the first time in my life, I am seeing the private culture of one of my peers. The childhood bedroom Gary and I share is still very much that − a child's bedroom, filled only with the things our parents have curated for us. But here was a place distinctly *other*, filled to the brim with Craig's own tastes and growing personality. It's all very strange, and it conspires to make me feel even younger and dafter and uncooler than I am − no mean feat in 1979. 'Listen to this,' Craig says.

I sit down on the brown-cream shag carpet as he takes an album from a primary colours sleeve: red, blue and yellow with black Chinese-style lettering at the top, an image of a man on horseback looking at a corpse laid face down in the desert, red blood coming through the blue shirt. A pair of vultures or buzzards sit on the corpse, one of them pecking at the bloodstain on the man's back. The image is exotic, dangerous, *alien*. RAF John vaguely wonders if what we are about to do is even strictly legal. This, I already feel certain, is not going to be Acker Bilk. As if conscious of the wild, radioactive contents of the black plastic disc, Craig holds it very carefully, just his fingertips on the edges as he places it on the turntable. He gently places the needle in the groove and turns the volume up as far as it will go. Hum and crackle from the small speakers and then an *explosion* of noise, a shockwave, an absolute wall of guitars, banging on what I will eventually come to know is an E barre chord at the seventh fret. (Many years from this day Stuart Braithwaite from Mogwai will tell me − and Christ he'd know − that this is undoubtedly 'the loudest chord on the entire guitar'.) The guitars, I will also learn in due course, were recorded by producer Sandy Pearlman over the course of five months and three different recording studios, at Sarm West in Notting Hill, at the Automat in San Francisco and, finally, at the Record Plant in New York City.

But I don't need to know any of this now. Because the singer is gabbling –

'Well, I just got back and I wish I never leave now . . .'

But he's singing it so fast, so desperately, that the words are tumbling over themselves in a mad, insane fever, coming out as – *'welllllahjus-gohbackannahwishahnevahleaveahnow'*.

I am transfixed in seconds. Within minutes, changed forever.

If you watch Taylor Hackford's 1987 Chuck Berry documentary *Hail! Hail! Rock 'n' Roll*, there is a moment where Keith Richards tries to explain the impact Berry's music had on him as a teenager. Lost for words, Keith kind of drifts off in reverie, tracing a shape in the air with his cigarette as he says 'It was just . . . the *sound* that came off that needle.' Bob Dylan has described how, as a little boy, sitting on the floor of his parents' house in Hibbing, Minnesota, he'd turned on the big mahogany radiogram and heard Bill Monroe singing 'Driftin' Too Far From Shore' and that the sound of the record 'made me feel like I was somebody else . . . like maybe I was born to the wrong parents'. John Lennon said that when he heard Elvis for the first time 'my head just turned', and I often picture this happening like Navin R. Johnson's in Steve Martin's *The Jerk*: his head going around in a complete 360 when he's told the value of that cheque. This was all happening to me now, in a three-bedroom council house in Castlepark, in September 1979. The smell of paraffin and joss sticks, the late-summer, late-afternoon sunshine coming in the window and 'Safe European Home' blasting out of Craig's stereo, telling me that everything I know is wrong.

Fuck Geoff Love.

Fuck German classes.

Fuck golf.

Fuck the RAF.

All of it, the tiny personality I'd been trying to assemble, blown away in the three minutes and fifty-one seconds it took to get from that first rush of guitars to the singer stuttering the word 'Rudy' over and over. We listen to it again. And again. And then the whole album. And then the album they made before this one: three men scowling in an alleyway, a slash of black-and-white photography on military green. Now this record even has a song on it that specifically says '*I hate the RAF.*' This was beginning to feel personal, like a taunt. Craig explains everything to me. The band were formed by the men in the picture above us, Mick Jones and Joe Strummer. They are childhood friends who grew up together in Brixton – which is a place in London – and they even wrote a song together about their childhood friendship called 'Stay Free'. It will be years before I learn that all of this – aside from the fact that Brixton is indeed in London – is utter cobblers. That Strummer and Jones didn't meet until they were in their twenties and were no more childhood friends than a couple of contestants yoked together on *The X Factor*. But no matter. I am *gone*. There is an aphorism about love, about its arrival with the twinned questions: '*Is it you? Is it now?*' Because the timing must be right. If the timing is right, it can be almost anyone. So it goes with your first musical crush. I am ripe to fall. Thirteen years old, roiling with hormones, the sound of the guitars stacked to the ceiling on *Give 'Em Enough Rope* speaking to every teenage molecule fizzing and raging inside me. By the end of the year The Clash will be the best band in the world and Craig will be my best friend. I will soon turn fourteen and will make a momentous decision.

I am going to buy an electric guitar.

Automatic Gay Bogs

Gary arrives at big school in August 1980, and duly begins experimenting with punk rock too. And, it must be said, he comes to it more naturally than me. His face lends itself more easily to the scowl. There's the crew cut and mohair sweater he adopts. And, perhaps most importantly, at twelve, he already has the 'fuck you' attitude down cold.

As Gary arrives at his teens, a tension begins to make itself felt between him and dad. On the one hand, he and Gary will kick the football around the back garden. Gary will join dad in the garage, over the workbench, copying him, hammering nails into bits of wood torn from the fish crates our nanny gets her haddock delivered in. They like the same TV shows and the same food: mince and tatties and baked beans stirred together into a kind of pink pulp that sends me – the latent ponce – running from the room in disgust. And yet there's something in Gary that won't be tamed. When caught in the wrong, I am fast to make with as eloquent a rationale/apology as I can. When berated over a poor report card, I will hang my head and vow to do better. Gary will shrug. Sneer. Scowl. He'll just say, 'Lee us alane.' He doesn't care about school. For dad, a blacksmith's son who became an electrician, who places a premium on the idea of education, this attitude becomes increasingly hard to take.

Gary's peer group grows at school, filling out with a crew of harder, wilder kids. Mine pretty much begins and ends with Craig. While my parents are puzzled by my burgeoning interest in punk rock, they are not yet alarmed. In fact, one Saturday afternoon, mum comes home from Ayr market with presents: some punk badges for me and Gary. One is pink with a pair of boot prints stamped on it in black along with the stark legend 'POGO ON A MOD'. This terrible call for violence is very much the 'My Ding-A-Ling'/'Laughing Gnome' of punk badges and it still gives me enormous pleasure, a lifetime later, to picture mum peering over the rows of badges on a stall at Ayr market before carefully selecting 'POGO ON A MOD'. Gary takes it, pinning it on his mohair sweater next to the 'VICIOUS BURGER' one he already carries off with aplomb. My parents sense no danger yet because I really am that most lamentable of creatures: a 'plastic' punk. It is about the worst insult that can be levelled at you at school. Remove a few badges and the Damned 'Smash It Up' armband I buy at Virgin Megastore in Glasgow – and which I only take from my pocket and slip on when I am a safe distance from the house – and I'd still pass for the old Partridge me. I am desperately trying to lose my side parting and briefly experiment with a crew cut like Gary's, but with far less success – I look like a grinning football with a layer of peach fuzz.

Once my hair grows back in enough, armed with a picture of Joe Strummer clipped from the *NME*, I boldly head downtown to George the Barber's, accompanied by a school friend, Alan Patterson. Of course, this being the dawn of the 80s, making it roughly 1962 in Ayrshire, George's was never referred to as 'George the Barber's'. It was 'Poofy George's'. It was unclear to me whether this was because George – who was certainly camp – was genuinely homosexual or because hairdressing was obviously a profession only for homosexuals. Similarly, the fish-and-chip shop where I received my beating a couple of years earlier, Mama's, was universally referred to as 'Black Mama's', as, at one point in its history, it had been owned by an African-Caribbean woman. Once within the walls of Black Mama's you might order a 'darkie's walloper and chips': a black pudding supper. The Chinese restaurant, the Loon Fung, was 'the Wan Lung'. And, naturally, it was only referred to as a 'Chinese' restaurant in the phone book, with my mother and brother both persisting with 'Chinky' well into the twenty-first century, despite the howls of protest from Linda and me, the family PC brigade. Years later, on a visit home from London, I am changing to go out for the night and have rung the Wan Lung to order a chow mein. The doorbell chimes and I start coming downstairs with the money. Mum beats me to the punch and I watch in horror as she takes the steaming bag off the – very clearly Chinese – delivery boy and cheerfully sings the words *'JOHN! THAT'S YER CHINKY!'* right into his face.

The public toilets next to the Wan Lung are known as 'the Gay Bogs'. Again, I was uncertain whether they really were a locus of flaming cottaging, or whether it was just assumed that any public toilet was guaranteed to be a cauldron of homosexual activity. At some point the reeking brickwork of the Gay Bogs is demolished and replaced by a modern, coin-operated robo-toilet. The new structure is immediately christened 'the Automatic Gay Bogs'. 'Why the hell are you calling the toilets that?' mum asks, having overheard Gary using the term.

''Cause it's where the poofs hang oot, maw!' Gary replies, always thrilled with how far he can push the envelope with mum. 'Aw that pure bent fur the rent way, man!'

'Gary! Language!' mum barks automatically, before adding, thoughtful, worried now, 'In *Irvine*?'

This perversion was surely an import of the Glasgow people too. A true innocent in such things, mum will be astonished when Rock Hudson's AIDS-related death is announced and will later struggle to comprehend the homosexuality of Freddie Mercury and George Michael, both of whose music she quite liked. At the end of the 90s, we will be watching TV when the video for 'Outside' comes on. 'Linda used to love him as well,' mum sighs. 'I just cannae believe he's . . .' Just before the word 'gay' can clatter from her mouth, we cut to George in cop-drag, suggestively wielding a truncheon as he dances in the mirror-balled public toilet, in some fabulous, deranged Automatic Gay Bog of the future.

'Yeah,' I say. 'We can close the book on this one, mum.'

So, at one point in 80s Irvine, in a holocaust of language undoubtedly stunning today, you could get a trim at Poofy George's, grab a darkie's walloper and chips from Black Mama's and pay a visit to the Automatic Gay Bogs on your way home.

In the barber's, George looks quizzically at the photo, at Strummer's impeccable DA, and proceeds to give me a short back and sides which he then plasters flat across my scalp with lotion. I can see the horror unfolding in the mirror – the fact that my moon features are not responding as well to this treatment as the chiselled bone

92

structure of Strummer or Jones. I realise that George is getting close to finishing and that things are not going to get any better. I look, at best, like a youthful Hitler and I begin to slowly turn bright red. Finally, George whips the apron off in *'VOILÀ!'* fashion and swivels me around in the chair to face the rest of the shop – a crimson Mitre 5 with hair plastered across its dome like Lord Snooty from the *Beano*. Alan Patterson *collapses* with laughter. Even the benign, elderly stranger sitting next to him looks up from his newspaper and simply emits a low whistle through his teeth before saying, 'Jesus Christ, son.'

Not an auspicious start to The Punkification of John Niven.

And it is a side parting of the very soul I am trying to change. Although I have packed the ATC in, I am still very much doing my homework, and the habit of thrusting your hand up Martin Prince-style when the teacher asks a question is hard to break. I know it's not very punk to, like, know stuff, but I can't seem to help it. Gary has no such qualms. He doesn't seem to care as his report cards spiral down and just shrugs when dad tells him that if he doesn't 'buck his ideas up' at school he's going to end up 'on the bins', working in refuse collection being very much dad's bleakest assessment of your prospects. For me, the thought of being a binman is so appalling that I redouble my efforts, cracking the books even as I pay lip service to 'anarchy'. I am still a wall hugger at school.

And here comes Gary, striding down the middle of the corridor, riding at the head of his men, laughing and shouting.

Gallus.

* * *

Sheila Ferguson at school says her big brother is selling an electric guitar for fifteen pounds, including an amplifier, and I agree to the deal sight unseen. I am fully expecting it to look like the guitar Mick Jones plays – what I don't yet know is called a Gibson Les Paul – but when the guy drops it off at our house I am horrified to be confronted by a big cherry sunburst semi-acoustic, with F-holes in it like a violin and a big metal bar that makes the strings go all wongy when you move it up and down. This is obviously a very un-punk guitar, and I carry it somewhat shamefully in a black bin bag through the streets of Irvine to Craig's house in Castlepark, where his big brother tries to show us a few simple riffs and chords. I get a book from the library, Frederick Noad's *Playing the Guitar: A Self-Instruction Guide to Technique and Theory*. But it's about classical guitar, so complex that it might as well be in hieroglyphics. Gradually, I just about master a couple of the most basic riffs known to man: the three-note, one-string motif of 'Satisfaction', the rolling, three-note intro to 'Pretty Vacant'.

I am sitting at the bottom of the stairs one afternoon, where the echo comes nice off the Artex walls, cranking my pitiful repertoire out when Gary strolls by and cocks an ear.

'Ho, gayboy. Show us how tae dae that Pistols wan.'

He takes the huge, badly tuned guitar and I try and get his fingers into the right places, trying to guide his strumming hand to pick the open A string and then its octave on the G string. After maybe five minutes of thwanging and fumbling and *gahh-doinging* Gary simply hurls the guitar aside and storms off, denouncing the whole business as a 'load of pish'. This, in its own way, was much more authentically punk rock than me, hunched over my Frederick Noad. But hunch I must, because Craig has bought a bass – a Gibson SG copy – and we

94

have decided our band will be called 'Suspect Device', after the Stiff Little Fingers song, the Northern Irish proto-Clash outfit being our new obsession as we begin rehearsing out in dad's wooden garage, surrounded by jars of screws and nails, with canvas bags of ancient golf clubs in racks above us (niblicks and mashies and cleeks) and the coppery heat-smell of the valves in the amplifiers mixing with the smells of creosote and engine oil. Gary will occasionally burst in the door to tell us it's 'utter shite', or that we are 'bentshots'. We are in here, probably working up a number called 'Thatcher – Satan', when mum comes in to tell us we're missing the royal wedding on TV. Charles and Di. We couldn't care less. Would Strummer be watching the royal wedding? Would *Wattie Buchanan*? Would he fuck.

With the guitar, I finally find my tribe. Along with Craig there is Graham Fagen, Allan Carruthers, Keith Martin and Clinky – who are all in our rival punk band, Ground Zero – and Leishman and Andy Kerr and Skin and wee Tam. And as we all start to spend our nights playing records and drinking green cans of Kestrel lager in the small woodchip-papered bedrooms of corporation houses – the squeak of leather jackets and the smell of hair teased skywards with soap – suddenly the big school begins to lose some of its terror.

Shades: Birth of a Legend

'The shades from a pencil peer, pass around . . .'

Another party at Whyte Avenue. Me and Gary and David and Kevin are upstairs, tipsy on stolen red tins of McEwan's Export, the dark beer bitter on our tongues, that proud, laughing cavalier, tankard raised. Back then, pre-aluminium, the joint in the can was still made of bolted steel, as though it had been roughly hewn in a Glasgow shipyard. Music comes through the floorboards from below, the laughter of the grown-ups, dancing and singing. We're singing too, playing records up in the bedroom David and Kevin share. *'The shades from a pencil peer, pass around . . .'* It's a throwaway line in the song, it only happens once, it's not the chorus or even a refrain, so I don't know why we all keep singing that line from The Human League's current single 'The Sound Of The Crowd', over and over again. Just that one line. In the way of recurring jokes, it gets more hilarious the more we repeat it. *'The SHADES.'* Then there will be a pause, we'll talk about something else, and then someone will bellow it out again, even more vehemently this time, with strong, needless emphasis on the word 'shades'. I can't remember if it was because Gary was singing it more than the rest of us, if he was the one who kept bringing it up again and again, but however it happened that night in the summer of 1981, it happened. It stuck.

The nickname for the rest of Gary's life is handed to him by the Wilson boys: from that day on he is forever known as 'Shades'. Wee Shades. Shadesy-boy.

There's undeniable coolness to the new nickname, with its invocation of sunglasses. It also reflects something of Gary's manner, the nervy, darting-eyes way he carries himself sometimes as he becomes a teenager. Always up to something. Shady. Also, with shadiness in-built, there are the gangsterish, ducking-and-diving connotations. And, to my horror, Shades *likes* The Human League. He's recently left punk behind, his musical tastes in his thirteenth year beginning to skew more towards the mainstream, towards Spandau Ballet and Duran Duran, bands more in keeping with his new friendship group at school. These are the boys who wear Pringle, whose waffle jumpers are tucked into their stonewashed jeans, with grey leather slip-on shoes, their hair in semi-mullets, perms and heavy wedges. Gold chains and sovereign rings. Of course, we, the punks, relentlessly mock the 'casuals', the 'neds', and their embarrassing taste in clothes and music. You'll have to imagine the heaviness of my sigh today, as I look at my brother's copy of The Human League's flawless, multi-million-selling, America-conquering masterpiece *Dare* sharing shelf space with one of the albums I favoured that year – *Another Kind Of Blues* by The UK Subs, in limited edition blue vinyl.

There's another big event at the end of the summer of '81, when my parents announce what is in hindsight a monumentally insane decision: they are going away for the weekend of 3 October, to visit friends

97

up north, near Aberdeen. They'll be taking Linda (now eight) with them but allowing Shades and I to stay at home.

With me in charge.

I am six months away from my sixteenth birthday and thought of as 'sensible'. Besides, our eighty-year-old grandmother still lives next door and will be popping in and out to keep an eye on us. What mum and dad have failed to account for is the extent to which punk rock has truly addled my mind. The scheme occurs to me one Saturday while we are practising out in the garage. We will, as they say, do the show right here.

The space is about thirty feet long and fifteen feet wide. If we clear every single tool, jar of nails, old set of golf clubs and spare tyre out, it might just hold around forty fifteen-year-olds. Worried about the pulling power of the nascent Suspect Device, we bring in Ground Zero, and the two bands get to work. Allan makes tickets, charging twenty pence to get in. Craig and Graham scavenge plastic crates from their milk rounds, and I get some big wooden boards from the skip behind dad's mall. These will be used to build the stage. Allan makes a set of lights using red, blue and green coloured bulbs and Craig spray-paints our backdrop: 'SUSPECT DEVICE', on a mushroom cloud, with the words 'NO FUTURE' at the base of the stem. We shift all fifty tickets (we're figuring on some no-shows) through word of mouth at school, netting a cool ten pounds between eight of us. We invest a quid of this in two bottles of Nigel Green's homebrewed 'cider' – closer to the urine of someone who had recently eaten an apple than traditional cider – to hire Big Davy Prentice as security. Big Davy is indeed so big that he can defend the stage simply by standing in the middle of the garage and touching each wall with his hands.

98

Saturday arrives. Our parents and Linda leave first thing, to return on Monday. Shades and I cheerfully wave them off from the front doorstep. Then, as in all good teen movies, as soon as the car disappears around the corner, I *run* for the phone. We set to it: clearing out dad's crap, building the milk-crate stage, putting up the lights and backdrops, setting up drums and amps. I have a cracked, faded, colour photograph from that afternoon: all eight members of the two bands, standing in the garage after we have completed these tasks. We are all grinning like lottery winners, dressed in our best punk finery, ecstatic that our mad scheme is so close to fruition. The image so powerfully captures the joy and hope of youth that now, more than forty years later, it is difficult for me to look at without pressure rising in my chest and trying to force itself out through my eyes. Night falls and the teenagers descend upon 143 Livingstone Terrace, packed to the gills with illicit carryouts: Strongbow and Skol and big green bottles of Cinzano and half-bottles of Smirnoff. About as many of them are here for the party (*'Niven's goat an empty, man!'*) as have come for the music, and things escalate in utterly predictable fashion. I am soon like a panicking junior officer under fire as every minute someone brings me fresh, terrible news: Big Sadie is performing a striptease for Shades in papa's shed, someone is pissing in the kitchen sink, someone has smashed the telephone in the hall, Big Rab is fingering wee Clare in my parents' bed. I'm wandering through the unfolding mayhem, trying to stop the worst of it, as prissily unnerved as Jagger at Altamont, when Craig finds me and screams, 'COME ON! WE'RE ON!'

It all passes fast in a blur of noise and chaos. The racket we make is surely hellish, but thirty-odd really pissed fifteen-year-olds crammed into a hot, confined space and confronted with loud noise respond predictably enough – they go nuts. Allan's homemade lights hot on your skin and sweating faces pogoing and then it's suddenly all over and I'm trembling as I drink a can of lager backstage, backstage being the square of concrete behind the garage. Finally, around 11pm, a plot device buried in the first act re-emerges in the third as my grandmother is finally roused from her television by the sound of the actual teenage rampage going on outside. Because people have spilled out of the house and garage and into the garden now, drinking and snogging and fingering and vomiting like they've just heard the four-minute warning we alluded to in our closing number. Nana appears with a broom, literally scourging the demons away.

'Go on, ye dirty wee buggers! Get oot o' here!'

Early the next morning, after a few hours' sleep, we all reassemble, get the gear out and return the garage and house to close to normal. In true *Risky Business*-style, the last amplifier has just been trundled around the corner on a skateboard as the Cortina pulls up.

I am, of course, immediately grassed up.

Not by Shades or nana, but by several of the neighbours. For I hadn't quite factored in that a punk rock concert inside the thin wooden walls of a garage might be overheard in some of the other terraced houses on the street. 'Worse than the bloody war,' is one of the reviews. I have 'let myself down' and am very much in the doghouse. I will 'never be given any responsibility again'. But, in a rare Shades-esque show of bravado, I don't care. The whole thing was worth it for those twenty minutes on stage, for the clarity they brought: for I now have an idea about what I might do with my life.

Shades Interruptus: Wanking,
Heavy Petting and Cunnilingus Fail

The family holiday in July 1981, to Siloth in Cumbria, as Brixton and Toxteth go up in flames and all summer long, everywhere, you hear the extremity of human sorrow in Terry Hall's voice as he tells us about bands being unable to play any more.

London and Liverpool are not the only things burning. The car journey from Ayrshire to the Solway Firth takes forever and, being fifteen, the rocking motion of the car does what it does to me as it snakes its way south. By the time we arrive at the holiday camp, I have what feels like a red-hot bar of titanium in my pants. It is the kind of erection I'll hear characterised years later, by a janitor at Glasgow University, as being so profound that 'a cat couldnae scratch it'. The moment we're in the door of the chalet, I head off to the bathroom where I lock the door and set about stealing a pauper's bliss . . .

Catcher's mitt of bog roll clamped in my left hand, just as things are about to resolve themselves unequivocally, The Worst Thing in the World happens: the door, which is on runners, a sliding job, begins to roll slowly and terribly open.

I have somehow failed to lock it.

Now, there are the horror stories from school, first-person accounts of this dread event. There was the lad frantically having a turn at himself when his mum strolled into his bedroom with some fresh laundry. The thrown clothes – 'HERE'S YOUR JEANS!' – and her tearful retreat. Or there was Stevie, off sick from school, the tempting box of Kleenex to hand, deciding to go for it in the living room, safe in the knowledge his mum was out in the back garden, when his dad entered, returning unexpectedly from work to find his first-born son resolutely about himself, pyjama trousers tightly banded between his ankles, snap-jawed in front of *Pebble Mill at One*. 'FOR GOD'S SAKE, STEVEN!' came the (to me) remarkably forgiving paternal response. 'THERE'S A BATHROOM FOR THAT SORT OF THING!'

And yet Stevie continued to live with his parents, which astonished me. Surely emigration or suicide were your only options in these scenarios? And here I was, my own reckoning dawning, titanium bar in hand, as I stared at the head-height spot of the opening door, where I was about to be confronted by the face of dad or – worse, oh, far worse – mum. But no. Nothing. I look down.

Shades, on the floor, leering horribly up at me, having lain on his belly and slowly pulled the door open.

'AHHHH! YA DIRTY BASTARD!' he screams delightedly.

I scramble to my feet, trying to pull my trousers up and aim a kick at his face at the same time. All to no avail. I fall down in a tangle as he runs off, overjoyed at his triumph.

When we return to school after the holidays, I see Shades leading a gang of his mates along the art corridor, their smirking intensifying as I approach. As I pass them, as if on cue, all of them simultaneously erupt and begin making the internationally recognised hand-pumping gesture at me, with Gary's madly happy face in the middle of the throng, his twinned fists working in the air, as if he is furiously pulling off two tumescent men standing on either side of him.

'HAHAHAHA! NIVEN – YA FUCKING WANKER!'

I am in my bedroom with Moira, my first serious girlfriend, and the petting is passing the stage frowned upon by public swimming pool signage of the time, edging into the zone labelled 'heavy', as heavy as the blood that lurches thick around my veins.

The sounds from downstairs, mum clanking pots in the kitchen, dad's laughter at something on TV. My trembling hand creeps inside her blouse and then over the satin cup of her bra, and then – incredibly, for the campaign to get here has taken *months* – it is slipping *inside* the material and then moving, seemingly unchecked, over actual flesh, the . . . this, it must be the *nipple* beneath my palm, her breath shortening, her body stiffening, her back beginning to arch as we–

The door flies open, a hell-figure bursting into the room.

We fly apart like electrons, Moira screaming, as Shades runs in, drops to his knees on the carpet and begins strumming an imaginary guitar as, to the tune of B.A. Robertson's recent 'off-beat' hit 'I Knocked It Off', he lustily sings –

'AH SOOKED THEM AFF! AH SOOKED THEM AFF! SHE WAS SITTING IN THE CORNER WI' HER BRASSIERE AFF!'

Before I can even react, his performance is finished and he is running back out of the room, his 'HAHAHAHAHAHAHAHA!' trailing behind him as he joins his cackling pals on the landing.

'NO WAY, MAN!' one of them shouts.

'AH DID IT!' he shouts ecstatically.

Moira buttons up her blouse and begins searching for her coat and shoes as I contemplate the kind of colossal strategic setback perhaps only fully known to, say, the German 6th Army in the winter of 1941.

A typical Saturday night of the time.

Craig's dad, being divorced, being single, is going out, handing us an 'empty'. Well, big brother Steven will be around, but he's fine with us and tends to hang out in his room with his friends, listening to their hippie music.

Craig and I begin our evening by loitering outside the Three Craws, the nearest pub to Castlepark. (It's actually called the Ravenspark Arms, but is never referred to as such, the mural of the three ravens picked out in black-on-white tiles that covers its front wall giving it the local name.) We lurk until a likely candidate approaches and then one of us asks the big question . . .

'Hey, mister, gaunnae get us a carryout?'

There are some boys we know who, at fifteen, are already able to swagger into an off-licence and get served. We are not among them. When we score our order is always the same: four cans of Bass Special, a quarter-bottle of Smirnoff for Craig and a quarter-bottle of Whyte & Mackay for me. I actually still hate the taste of whisky, but mixed with enough SodaStream lemonade, I can get it down. I buy it because that's what my dad drinks, just as Craig drinks vodka because his dad does, your alcohol preferences on the west coast of Scotland being as strongly inherited as your Labour politics. After a while a cheerful middle-aged man takes our money, brings back the goods, and we trudge back to Craig's house and lie on the carpet in the living room, getting drunk as we listen to records until, having finished our cans

104

and quarter-bottles, having taken as much gazing at Pennie Smith's *The Clash: Before & After* book and listening to *Sandinista!* and *Sound Affects* as man can take, Craig and I go out for a drunken weave through the streets of Irvine.

Gradually, as a light rain begins to fall, we wind our way across the wall that separates the Castlepark estate from old Irvine (not enough of a Berlin Wall for my mum's liking) and on into band three of the town, not far from my house, where we bump into Karen, Diane and Senga – girls we know from school. They too have been having their Saturday night cans and quarter-bottles. We stand around making small talk, the girls tugging on Consulates, the smoke drifting up through the raindrops sparkling in the orange lozenges of the streetlights. After a bit, Karen takes me by the arm, leads me a little way off, and, with much giggling and glancing over, lets it be known that Senga likes me. She *likes* me likes me. I look over to see Senga, who is in a couple of my classes, talking away to the others, her back to us, drawing fiercely on her menthol. She has dark curly hair and her red jeans are as tight as a second skin. 'ANTMUSIC FOR SEXPEOPLE' reads one of the badges on her black leather bomber jacket and this seems a most promising omen indeed. Senga comes from the Winton Road area, one of the rougher enclaves of the town, and isn't the kind of girl I'd have pictured taking an interest in someone like myself, but the list of those who do is short and undistinguished. In my heart I am still very much a Sandy kind of guy, but sometimes life puts a Rizzo in your path. So, it's very much a no-brainer when Karen opens the door to romance by asking if I'd be interested in taking a stroll 'up the garages' with Senga.

The drizzle is falling harder as the two of us wander off the main street and down a potholed, waterlogged side road between two terraces of council houses. There are battered wooden garages lining either side of the track, some with tarpaulin covering their broken roofs, the rain fairly sizzling off the tarp. She takes me by the hand and leads me between two of them. (And right about now, somewhere south of us, in Manchester, there is an aspiring lyricist who could make a pretty good fist of this kind of scenario.) We kiss, and it's immediately wilder than any encounter I've had so far: tongues plunging, my hands in those soaking dark curls, her burying her face in my neck, nibbling and sucking and biting. We are drunk and in the wild, with no parents clattering around below, no Gary crouching outside the door, squinting through a crack, cocked and ready with a well-turned parody lyric. Quickly, I'm scrabbling at the button on those red jeans, and then they're popping open and my fingers are plunging into an altogether different tangle of dark curls and there is no resistance, no resistance at all. It is unbelievable. *Antmusic for sexpeople.* With hammering heart I realise that, more than anything in life, I need, with maximum urgency, to *see* it and, before I quite know what I'm doing, I'm dropping to my knees, down there on the soaking gravel, with the smell of wet creosote all around, tugging that crimson denim down, the white of her belly in the black night, as I push my face into her, burying myself in it. Senga grabs me by the hair and tugs my head back with a fierceness I take to be passion. Until I look up into her enraged face.

'WHIT YE DAEING, NIVEN? FUCK SAKE! IT STINKS DOON THERE!'

Ah, my Senga. '. . . *while thy willing soul transpires, at every pore with instant fires, now let us sport us while we may . . .'* Sadly, I am still three years away from getting to grips with Andrew Marvell's

'To His Coy Mistress', so this entreaty is not yet available to me. She pushes me off and I fall back into a puddle, to watch her strut off between the garages, buttoning up as she marches back into the cold, wet night, shaking her head, horrified at my perversion. My pleasures, like Marvell's, are doomed to remain untorn through the iron gates of life.

The next morning, Sunday, I freeze in terror before the bathroom mirror as I discover that, inconclusive though it may have been, the encounter with Senga has left its mark upon me: the huge, livid bruise on my neck, fading from its Bordeaux centre into the yellow of ancient parchment at the edges.

I frantically apply the famous remedy: grinding toothpaste into the afflicted area. To no avail. Only one thing could possibly make the situation worse. And it duly arrives as soon as I emerge distraught from the bathroom onto the tiny landing and walk straight into him.

'Whit . . . whit's that oan yer neck?' Shades asks, immediately delirious with excitement as I try to barge past him, his finger pointing at my neck.

'Is that . . . is that *A LOVEBITE?* HAHAHAHAHAHAHAHAHA! Whit total, utter midden gave *you* a fucking nookie badge, ya bawbag? HAHAHAHAHAHAHAHA!'

I slam my door. *Oh, baby, I'm dreaming of Monday.*

Which arrives promptly. *Ring ring, 7am.* And, in the end, all the tightly buttoned-up shirt collars and all the toothpaste in Ayrshire wouldn't have mattered. Because Gary duly tells the whole school, his finger joining the now familiar pointing forest of them as I edge, face burning, along the corridor. And it fast becomes clear, from the content of some of the taunts, that it is not only Gary who has betrayed me.

The fickle Senga has cruelly played her part too . . .

'NIVEN GOAT A LOVEBITE AFF SENGA MCALLISTER UP THE GARAGES! HE TRIED TAE LICK HER FANNY SO HE DID, MAN! GADS O' FUCK! HAHAHAHAHAHAHA!'

The grave is a fine and private place indeed, Andrew.

The Socks of Paul Simonon

The news, in the *NME*, at the beginning of 1982, blows our tiny minds – The Clash are coming to play Scotland on the *Combat Rock* tour. Not only that, they are coming to play *in our actual town*. At the Magnum Leisure Centre down the harbour.

And not only that, the show is scheduled for 1 May, my sixteenth birthday. *The Clash*, in our town, *on my birthday*. (In hindsight I can see that the date was fortuitous for reasons beyond the birthday co-incidence. Just a year or so earlier and I probably wouldn't have been allowed to go. Much more than a year later, and you'd have had to coax me down there with red-hot pokers, having decided by then that The Clash were 'rockist' and passé.)

Then the unthinkable happens. We open the *NME* to see that Strummer has vanished. He's done a runner, apparently concerned about 'the role of the artist in our bubblegum pop culture' – and the entire tour has been postponed, perhaps to be cancelled altogether. I am inconsolable.

Finally, Joe is found in Paris and – slack ticket sales having mysteri-ously picked up following all the publicity around his disappearance – the tour is back on, with the Irvine show rescheduled for Thursday,

22 July. In a way this is even better as it's during the summer holidays. Suspect Device drummer Andy Kerr and I hatch a plan: we're going to go down there in the morning and hang around all day. The band will probably be there, we reason, getting their stuff set up. That takes ages. This we know. They might want a hand. We can hang out and get to know each other. Maybe show them around the town. Take them up the dug track. To the Pancake Place.

We arrive promptly at 10am on a scorching summer morning to find absolutely nothing happening. We go into the Magnum and have a Slush Puppie and hit the Asteroids machine. Watch the ice skating. We go for a walk along the harbour. Then back to the venue. Still nothing. We take a walk down the harbour. Go back. Finally, around lunchtime, trucks begin to pull up on the grass at the side entrance to the venue and a bunch of guys in their twenties – many of whom are sporting Mohawks – start hauling out huge stacks of speakers, lighting and staging rigs. We circle them at a distance, walking by casually in the hope that one of them will say, 'Hey, son, give us a hand with this.' Or, admittedly more unlikely, that one of them will grab me and utter the words that have triggered many a schoolboy fantasy – 'Mick couldn't make it. Do you know the songs, kid?'

Eventually we muster the courage to make eye contact with one of the crew. He's young, early twenties, shades, Mohawk, stripped to the waist, sweating in the heat and clearly very busy.

'Umm, excuse me. Do you need a hand?'

He looks at us – me just sixteen, Andy fifteen, nothing much on either of us – and just shakes his head before walking away with a mile of cable over one shoulder and half a PA system under the other arm. We notice another guy helping them, and, from a distance, he

110

looks familiar: a few years older than us, dark, curly hair, olive skin, Clash T-shirt and combat trousers. It dawns on me that it's a face I haven't seen in three years: Sergeant Pieroni, from Irvine Air Training Corps. I think about saying hello but I'm too intimidated. Besides, if he's now a Clash roadie, he might not thank me for saying, 'Hi, I haven't seen you since we were trying to get into the RAF.'

Our dance around the road crew continues through the afternoon, our nerve gradually increasing as we realise these guys are far too busy to take much notice of us. We get closer and closer to the side entrance to the sports hall, the loading dock. Inside we can see that the stage is being built, the speaker stacks going up on either side. The familiar black-and-yellow striped stage set is emerging, hung with combat netting. And then we're inside, hugging the breeze-blocked wall, staying about as far from the action as we can while still being in the same room. We're trying to look invisible and like we're absolutely meant to be there at the same time. And we're not the only ones; about a dozen other nervous youths lurk, all in their own homemade approximations of The Clash's *Combat Rock*-era stage wear: the band's look at the time being Vietnam chic as interpreted by the designer Joe Casely-Hayford, ours being Paddy's Market army surplus as interpreted by your mum, who would have to take the sleeves off.

To the left of the stage, guitars are now being taken out of cases and tuned. My heart leaps at the sight of Mick's pair of Les Paul Customs: one midnight black and one alpine white. And then there's Joe's battered Telecaster, the silver flash of the 'IGNORE ALIEN ORDERS' sticker glinting under the strip lighting of the sports hall, the same legend I'd seen for the first time on the poster in Craig's bedroom. On stage left, Mick's pair of Mesa Boogie amplifiers have

111

been set up on top of their pair of Marshall speakers, his space age rack of effects between the amps. Strummer's little Music Man combo and Simonon's enormous Ampeg bass rig sit stage right as you look at it. We edge closer to the stage, drawn by the red and orange lights glowing on the amps. It's perhaps difficult to explain to someone who doesn't know what it is to be a deranged sixteen-year-old fan of a rock and roll band, but it is thrilling for us to be just yards away from these things, for they are sacred objects to us. We have gazed at them for hours in photographs for nearly three years. I feel like Kenneth Clark in *Civilisation*, standing speechless with awe in front of Chartres cathedral.

But it's late afternoon and there's still no sign of the band. Every time a member of the crew walks close to us our hearts pound with the fear that we are finally about to be thrown out. Every time a new adult walks in through the big loading doors that open out onto the grass and sunshine of Irvine beach park we almost snap to attention, thinking that, now, surely, it must be them. And then Andy nudges me in the ribs.

Strummer and Simonon are walking in.

It is the first time I have ever seen famous people in the flesh. Their heads look absolutely enormous: Easter Island/Mount Rushmore affairs planted on tiny bodies. They look like cartoons of themselves. (I will experience this phenomenon several times in adult life: Mick Jagger, Vin Diesel, Sylvester Stallone, Noel Gallagher. It's standard-issue with very famous people and has to do with image/size displacement: suddenly being face-to-face with someone very familiar to you, but only from tiny photographs and TV screens.) Strummer is wearing Raybans and is deep in conversation with a man we recognise from

Pennie Smith's book as Kosmo Vinyl, their press spokesman. They do not hang around, the pair of them disappearing through a door at the far end that I know leads to the squash courts. Are they getting a quick game in before the show? Paul Simonon stops however. He perches himself up on top of the wooden crash barrier that has been built in front of the stage and starts to sign autographs and chat to a group of fans far bolder than us. Or, as it seems to me, far more gauche. Even so, Andy and I gradually creep towards the huddle around Simonon, who is chatting away amiably in that familiar Brixton bass rumble, talking about the tour, about how much he likes Scotland, about how he's sorry the band haven't played here in so long. Someone compliments the tattoo on his bicep – the rear end of a yellow cab pulling away from a skyscraper. He says he had it done last year, in New York. He's sitting up on the wooden platform, his crotch at about our shoulder height, with his legs dangling down. I am *desperate* to insert myself into the conversation and, for some reason, I find I am looking at his socks. Now, we are of an age where we, and all of our friends, wear only plain, white sports socks. Anything else, anything black or grey or navy or ribbed, reeks to us of 'dad'. Simonon, I see, is wearing *brown* socks. Even worse, there are little diamond patterns down the side. There is a lull in the conversation. Clearly none of us wants Simonon to leave, we're living the dream here. Someone has to do something to keep the conversation going. And I've got just the thing. Obviously, I'm not about to ask him where he got his tattoo, or for his autograph, or anything idiotically fanboy like that. No, no, that won't do.

'Hey, Paul,' I say, all casual and matey. 'They're really horrible socks.'
Silence.

Utter total silence.

Simonon looks at me, his blue eyes cold, his gaze as blank and pitiless as the sun. My face begins to burn as the bass player of The Clash – a man who has routinely topped polls of 'the coolest people in rock', whose straddled, possibly brown be-socked feet as he smashes his Fender Precision bass on the cover of *London Calling* will become one of the most iconic images in all of rock and roll – glances briefly at his socks before looking me up and down: a crimson-ball-faced idiot in thrift-shop combat gear, before he turns back to the others and says, 'Anyway, cheers, lads. See you later, yeah?' He hops down and strolls off the same way Joe and Kosmo went.

The other Clash fans turn and look at me in utter disbelief. There is muttering and shaking of heads as they all disperse off into the hall, the words 'prick', 'fanny' and 'wee dick' patently audible.

'Aye, John,' Andy Kerr says to my burning face. 'Good one.'

Thankfully our lingering manages to survive my appalling behaviour. Indeed, we are even rewarded for it when the band soon reappear and make their way onstage to run through their sound check. At this point all pretence of cool leaves the building. No one is hanging onto the brown brick walls any more. We all emerge, like timid creatures creeping from the forest to the watering hole, and stand right in front of the stage. We cannot believe it. We are about to be treated to a mini-concert for a select handful. Strummer straps on his black Telecaster and Simonon his Precision as Terry Chimes climbs behind the kit. But . . .

There is no Mick Jones.

His mountain of amplification sits silent as the three-piece Clash play through skeletal, instrumental versions of two *Sandinista!* tracks,

'The Call Up' and 'The Leader'. And then – that's it. They're off. Strummer doesn't even open his mouth to sing! Now today, of course, you understand that – forty dates into a hundred-and-fourteen-date tour that began in Japan in January and will end in Jamaica in November – old Joe was simply preserving his voice for the show. But where the hell was Mick? We discuss it endlessly after the trio leaves the stage, as the road crew ushers everyone out into the sunlight. At this point in our lives, we still assumed that the band all lived together, in one big house like The Beatles in *Help!* Was he ill? Would they be doing the gig as a three-piece? It'd sound really bare and empty if it was like the sound check. Jesus Christ, maybe that schoolboy fantasy would come true after all. I'd have to smooth things over with Paul first, obviously. I picture rushing home to fetch my Kay Les Paul copy. And then, after the phenomenal success of my stand-in, the tears and anguish from my parents as I tell them, yes, I know I'm a bit young, but, the thing is, I'm moving to London to join The Clash. The anguished drink Mick and I will have – Malibu and Coke for me – as he wishes me all the best and tells me there's no hard feelings.

What we couldn't know that afternoon was that Strummer and Simonon *loathed* Mick Jones at this point. That the band were barely on speaking terms and were travelling separately whenever possible.

Come showtime we are crammed right down the front, sandwiched up against that wooden crash barrier, between Strummer and Jones' mic stands, a few yards along from where Sockgate took place. It is already *boiling* in here as, finally, the lights go down, Morricone's entrance music comes up. There's a roar and, despite my fantasies, a wave of relief floods through me as Mick Jones runs onto the stage with the rest of the group. And they really do *run* onto the stage, hitting it with an urgency I have never seen a band do before or since. Strummer is in red, Simonon in yellow and Jones in olive green. 'Good evening, ladies and gentlemen,' Joe says. 'London calling to the faraway towns.' With that, on the downbeat, Jones and Simonon both simultaneously leap five feet into the air and it begins. It is *deafening*. I am perhaps fifteen feet in front of Mick's wall of amplification: ten 12-inch speakers running at phenomenal volume. He stomps on round black pedals taped to the floor, causing tiny red lights on the FX units to blink and flash on and off, the needles on the illuminated VU meters in the top left corner of the two units tipping crazily over into the red, his guitar drenched in reverb and chorus, echoing and phasing and flanging all at once, screaming and rushing like the teenage blood in your veins. The difference in sheer volume from the sound check is incredible; it makes the (many) fillings in my Ayrshire teeth rattle. My ribcage crushes inwards. You can feel the sound moving the air, pushing your hair back, the bass drum like repeated punches in the stomach. Sweat is soon pouring down Strummer's right arm, running off his little finger in a stream and pooling on the stage next to his constantly pumping leg. I am so close I can see that their guitar leads have white plastic end caps with the word 'WHIRLWIND' stamped on them in black. Steam is pouring off the crowd in great clouds and roadies pass plastic gallon canisters of water into the front rows and spray them over us. I understand quickly that this is the greatest rock and roll show I have ever seen. I am some years away from understanding it is the greatest one I will ever see. They end with 'Clampdown' and come back on for two encores, finishing, twenty-six songs and nearly two hours later, with 'Garageland'.

Utterly spent, soaked to the skin with sweat, we meet up with Keith, Graham, Craig and Allan and we walk home together along the harbourside, the summer moon a perfect circle on the dark water as we sing 'Garageland' and 'Complete Control' and 'Stay Free', as we obsess over moments from the gig. (The following year, as I get to know Sergeant Pieroni – Basil – better, he will tell me about what went on backstage after the show. About the party and hanging out with the band and the endless free beer and spliffs and getting his hair cut into a Mohawk by Kosmo Vinyl.) The night has doubled down on everything I've been thinking since I bounded down off that milk-crate stage in our garage the previous autumn. And, walking home along Irvine harbour on that extraordinary summer evening, ears ringing, my life plan aged sixteen coalesces.

1) Learn how to play guitar properly.

2) Play real gigs.

3) Get in the *NME*.

4) Go on tour and play gigs every single night, in the places you read about in the *NME*, exotic places like Manchester and Sheffield and Leicester.

Places like London . . .

Some Wee Fud

Along with the metamorphic, the quotidian.

Few things create as much excitement in our house as the arrival of the new Grattan catalogue. As small children Gary and I would flip past the lingerie pages in seconds to spend hours basking in the carnival colours of the toy section. Inevitably, as puberty advanced, these proportions were exactly reversed. Sometimes, too, the Grattan catalogue would provide for our fashion needs. In 1982 it is the place where I get my first biker's jacket, a must-have item for the provincial punk rocker. For the last couple of years, I have been making do with a black, imitation-leather bomber jacket. I have been begging and lobbying for the real thing, but they retail at fifty to sixty pounds. I might as well have been asking for an actual motorbike. And then I find a real, black leather biker's jacket in the Grattan catalogue: it is a bargain thirty-six pounds, just about in the price range that, if I combine birthday and Christmas presents and chip in some pocket money, could be doable. And we can pay it off in instalments, mum! After a couple of months of listening to crap like this, mum caves in and, four to six weeks later, I am tearing open the packaging.

Finally, I'm a real punk, Geppetto.

And then my stomach is sinking, my face flushing hot.

On closer inspection, I see what could not be seen in the catalogue photograph, that the jacket is *patchworked* together, the stitching clearly visible, Frankenstein-style. It is made up of hundreds of small squares of leather stitched together. The thirty-six-quid price tag was a bargain for a reason. But I have begged for this jacket so much that I cannot possibly show any disappointment. I duly set off for school in it, close to tears all the way, fully knowing what I am going to be greeted with the second I walk into the playground, eyes downcast, my cheeks already warming, limbering up for the full burn, for the forest of pointing fingers and the joyful, outraged screams that do indeed instantly greet my arrival . . .

'CHECK THE STATE O' NIVEN'S BIKER JACKET, MAN!'

'IT'S AW STITCHED THEGITHER!'

'HAHAHAHAHA, YA PLASTIC, YE! *YA PLASO!*'

It is worse than Nookiebitegate. Than Jawsgate.

The other significant purchase from the Grattan catalogue around this time is more sinister. Shades and I have long marvelled over the pages of air pistols and air rifles, filled with the intoxicating thought that perhaps, when I was over the legal age of fourteen, one of the guns could perhaps be ours. Again, after much begging and pleading, mum and dad cave in and consent to the purchase of a Milbro G10 .177 air pistol. But dad has a respect for firearms born of his time in the armed forces and he lays down strict rules . . .

We are to use it only for paper targets in the garden.

It is never to be taken out of the house.

Most importantly – you never, ever, point a gun at someone.

Yes, yes, of course, we agree.

The pistol is matt black and looks exactly like a Colt .45 automatic. In reality the weapon is grossly underpowered and hopelessly inaccurate, and our delight at blasting paper targets in the garage quickly wanes. Soon we are plinking at cans and bottles, but the gun is too feeble to break glass or even puncture aluminium at a distance. We progress to trying to shoot sparrows and seagulls: the former proves impossible – too small and fast – and the latter impervious. I score a direct hit on a huge, proud gull that is shouldering its way around the back garden like a heavyweight boxer. The pellet bounces uselessly off its massive Scottish chest and it looks at me coolly – as though it is saying, *'Is that aw ye've goat, ya wee dick?'* – before flying off. Soon enough we are breaking all of dad's commandments: taking potshots at each other's arses around the house and smuggling the pistol out to go up the woods with my mates.

A Saturday afternoon and a bunch of us are strolling through Castlepark with Gary in tow. Coming along on his bike on the other side of the road is wee Davy Grant. Now, we have nothing in particular against this kid, he's just some wee fud. Gary happens to be carrying the air pistol at the time, sticking out of his belt like in the movies.

'Hey, Shades,' someone says. 'Bet ye cannae hit him.'

Shades has the gun out and up before the challenge has finished issuing. I don't even warn him off, because I'm thinking the same thing everyone else is – *no fucking chance*. It's a shot of over fifty yards, at a moving target in a fair breeze, with a weapon you can't hit a can at ten paces with. Shades tightens his finger on the trigger as Davy approaches on the other side of the road, his tongue jutting out in concentration, one eye closed, the pistol in a proper two-handed shooter grip.

CLACK.

Davy comes flying off his bike, rolling around on the ground, rubbing his neck as he screams '*eye-yah-eye-yah-eye-yah!*' It is, by any measure, a feat of incredible marksmanship. And Gary is once again at the centre of a cheering throng of older boys. Wee Davy – who isn't seriously hurt, the pellet hasn't even broken the skin – shouts and curses, fist raised as he picks up his bike and charges off, vowing revenge. We are just five or ten minutes along the road, still laughing, when the police van appears. It passes, slows, turns around and pulls up beside us. Two policemen get out.

'Open your jackets, boys.'

A resident has called to report boys shooting at people with a pistol. Gary opens his jacket to show the butt protruding from his waistband. He gamely attempts a 'how did that get there?' expression. As soon as our names are taken down and they establish that we are brothers, the two of us are being hustled into the back of the van, the Black Maria. In the back, on a wooden bench, stomach churning, I look at Gary.

'Ye aw said Ah couldnae hit him!'

The police van pulls up at our house. The shame, the burning agony of having the law on the doorstep of John Niven Snr. The manager of the shopping mall. The cops – one of them knows dad – explain what has happened, that Gary has shot at a boy with an airgun, and dad apologises while mum cries softly behind him. The policemen are content to leave it at a warning. They hand dad the air pistol and head off. The front door closes. Dad turns around and launches a fist into Gary's upper arm, driving him back along the hall. He is *enraged*. It starts with that dead arm and then a flurry of flat hands to his backside, as he would have done when we were small, but much harder now, smacking him as he shouts in time with each blow – 'AH TELT YE! AH TELT YE! AH TELT YE NO TAE TAKE THAT BLOODY GUN OUT OF THE HOUSE!' But Gary's not that small now, at fourteen. He isn't going to take this. Struggling to get free, he shouts back at dad – 'LEE US ALANE! LEE US ALANE!' And then, incredibly, 'FUCK OFF!'

'WHAT DID YOU SAY TO ME?'

I don't know who is more astonished he's said this, me or mum or dad or Gary himself. Dad's fist becomes bunched as he punches Gary again on the leg, on the arms, driving him further along the hall, into the kitchen. His belt comes off as Gary goes down, cowering on the kitchen floor while dad flails at him. He looks up at mum, appealing for clemency, for mercy. But there is none. I watch, behind the three of them, somehow, remarkably, escaping the same punishment. Dad grabs the air pistol from the hall table and charges out onto the back step. He fetches an axe from the garage and smashes it to pieces, its black metal casing breaking open, sparks flying as he misses sometimes, the axe glancing off the concrete step, springs and levers flying out under the fury of his blows, and Gary sprawled wailing and crying on the brown linoleum floor of the kitchen.

Where was I in all of this? Like in the caravan, with nana, I stood there, looking on while Gary took it. Why wasn't I getting it too? It was my air pistol. I was there with him. I'm two years older, surely the one in charge? I'm not getting it because I know how to play the game. Because, from the moment we came in the door, I stood there meekly, subservient, penitent, humble. Close to tears. It was that 'fuck off' that did it, more than the offence, even more than the police coming to the door.

122

As you make your way through what the literature has to say about hitting children, you are repeatedly confronted by the same conclusions. That it turns them into angry, resentful adults with psychological and emotional problems. That, counterintuitively, the more physical punishment children receive, the more defiant they become. The poorer their relationships are with their parents, the more likely they are to hit a partner or spouse. The more prone they are to mental health problems. To anxiety, depression and substance abuse. But this was the early 80s in working-class Scotland. *Everyone's* parents hit them. For most it was a spanking or a slap or the belt. Although, as we got further into our teens, you would hear terrifying stories of some of the bigger lads, the Tom Sellecks, the Big Rabs who faced off with their fathers in true fist fights, come-aheads, square goes.

At Ravenspark we have two tech teachers around dad's age, both called Milton. There's Big Milton and Wee Milton. Wee Milton is also known as Adventure Kit Milton, due to his belt crammed with tools and pouches. Back then the guys who taught the tech subjects – technical drawing, woodwork and metal work – tended to come from shop-floor backgrounds rather than academic ones. They could be pretty rough and ready. In woodwork one afternoon, Adventure Kit Milton is being harassed by two boys, one on either side of him, peppering him with questions – with 'Sir, sir, sir, sir, sir, sir, sir' – as he is trying to do something else, until, finally, he blows whatever tiny fuse he has. He punches one boy in the stomach, doubling him up, and grabs the second by his thick rug of hair and smashes his head several times off a metal cabinet. Today you picture the newspaper headlines, the sacking, the court case and the staggering sums of compensation. Back then, in 80s Ayrshire, Adventure Kit Milton just walked off and class went right on as normal.

One day, walking down the corridor, I am stopped by the other Milton – Big Milton – who enquires if I am related to John Niven senior. When I reply in the affirmative, he nods, pleased. 'Great wee football player in his day, your dad. Good golfer too. But' – and here he gave a low whistle through his teeth as he went misty-eyed, remembering something – 'he had some temper on him, so he did . . .'

'We got a letter from the school today, Henry . . .'

Jean Doole, the head of the English department, takes me under her wing, I think correctly suspecting that I am 'brupid': bright, yet still stupid. Gradually, I excel in English. An A at O-Level, then again at Higher, a band-one pass too, no less, right at the very top. I start reading outside the syllabus, and it is in the small library on the ground floor of school, in the spring of 1984, that I remember laughing, properly laughing out loud, at a line in a novel for the first time. The book is Heller's *Catch-22* and the line that ends me is: *'Major — de Coverley had a face so fearsome that no one had ever dared ask his first name.'* Alone at a table in the library, my face in my hands as the fit subsided, I flipped back to the title page and saw that, incredibly to me, the book had been published in 1961, five years before I was born. *Jesus*, the thought occurred to me, *imagine being able to do this to someone with something you wrote over twenty years ago?*

In the small, partitioned-off bedroom I start to spend my nights with books and records and my guitar, underlining passages, strumming chords, looking out the window at the lamppost that casts a tangerine

124

glow through the thin curtains and over the brown pebbledash houses at the junction of Livingstone Terrace and Dick Terrace, the street that runs north towards Castlepark.

Like Yossarian, I'm thinking, *how do I get out of here?*

But for Shades, it's all going in the other direction. The truancy officer arrives at our door. It transpires that Gary has been dogging the school. He's been forging mum's signature on an increasingly unconvincing series of sick notes and has not been for weeks.

Weeks.

He's been spotted downtown, hanging out in the amusement arcade, playing Frogger, Defender and Galaxian with his pals. Mum cries tears of shame. Dad is called at work. He comes home and is ready and waiting for Gary when he strolls in the door around 4pm, perhaps puzzled as to why the car is in the driveway so early, but basically secure in the belief that another successful day's deception is behind him, the boredom of the classroom dodged, a few high scores left proudly on a few screens, 'SHADES' dancing in brilliant graphics on the black background of space. I picture the whistle dying on his lips as he enters the living room to see dad standing there, breathing hard, belt already off. When I come home later, mum is quiet, still tearful, and dad is smouldering behind his clutched *Daily Record*. In the kitchen, in a whisper, Linda tells me what happened. Dad went *scripto*, thrashing at Gary with belt and then fists, pummelling him on the legs, the arms, his sides, until Gary was driven onto the carpet and went scuttling across the room on his hands and knees taking cover under the dining table, hanging onto one of the legs as dad tried to pull him out, mum and Linda wailing.

Finally, dad's super-fury burned itself out and Shades was sent to his room for the night unfed, dad's taunts about how he would end

125

up a bloody bum – on the bins or in the Bar-L – ringing in his ears. Later, after our near wordless, Garyless tea, I creep upstairs and softly ascend the metal ladder to the attic bedroom. He's on his single bed in the dark, turning away, turning his back to me as I come up through the trapdoor, not wanting me to see the sheen of dried tears on his face.

'Are you OK?'

No reply.

I had dogged the school myself of course. The odd morning, a stolen afternoon, the whole thing planned meticulously each time, alibis cross-referenced with pals, and all the time with my heart jammed in my throat, with the sense that I was taking the most incredible risk. The idea of doing it repeatedly, of doing it for weeks on end? You might as well have asked me to perform an armed robbery. I need to ask him.

'Shades, how did you think you'd get away with it?'

He doesn't speak or turn around. He just shrugs, a soft creak of the bedsprings as his shoulder blades work quickly up and down in the dark. What dad has failed to understand is that he is dealing with someone else now. The twelve-year-old Gary might not have taken these risks, but that guy is gone. The fourteen-year-old Shades is here.

And he doesn't do meek, or subservient, or penitent, or humble. He'll do what he likes and take whatever comes his way. Perhaps – and we'll throw in another movie reference, you'd have liked all these, Gary – Shades had now simply reached the same conclusion as the young Henry Hill, when he's faced with the consequences of his own truancy in *Goodfellas*: everybody takes a beating sometimes. The hardening of heart and hide. Dad's fists, bouncing pointlessly off him.

PART THREE

Wednesday, 1 September 2010

I pick up the gun while Linda screams at me to 'leave it alone!' It's a semi-automatic pistol, a Glock 17, heavy as a bag of sugar. Linda looks on, astonished and horrified and saying *'putitdownJohnputitdownJohn!'* as I thumb the catch to eject the magazine, which is empty, then pull the slide back to check the chamber, which is also empty. I let the slide snap back and dry-fire the pistol. *Click.* Linda looks at me, aghast.

If Gary and I had a competition for 'who has watched *Lethal Weapon* and *Die Hard* the most times?', it would have been a close-run thing. Like all idiot-boy obsessives who watch too many action films, you pick up on the hardware, on the lingo. As Shades would have told you, John McClane uses a Beretta 92FS, as did Martin Riggs of course. (Fifteen-shot magazine. Sixteen if you put one in the pipe.) By the time we get to *Die Hard 2*, as any fool knows, the bad guys are toting Glocks, and, pretty soon after, no one loved the Glock more than the drug dealer. On the trips I have begun to make to LA as a screenwriter in the last couple of years, a producer friend has taken me to a shooting range, where I have fired a Glock, among other handguns. Linda continues to watch as

I examine the weapon and confirm what I suspect – it's a replica, with a filled-in barrel, incapable of firing anything other than blank ammunition.

'What's he even doing with this?' Linda asks.

I put it in the carrier bag along with all the unpaid bills. We'll have to get rid of it somehow. As we leave the bedroom to go back downstairs, on impulse Linda opens the door of the hall cupboard. It's the kind of place you'd normally store towels and bed linen, but it's empty, bare, and the shelves have been removed. We notice a vertical line in the wood in the middle of the back wall. Linda presses it gently and it springs open – revealing a false cupboard behind the real one: a hidden compartment, most certainly built by our brother the carpenter. It's lined with tinfoil and empty too, save for a couple of flowerpots, and the unmistakable sage-and-oregano waft of weed. A tiny cannabis factory. We look at each other. The sword under the mattress, the replica handgun in the bedside drawer. Did he have these to hand just because he thought they were cool? (I can picture him sitting watching TV and playing with the pistol, racking the slide, ejecting the magazine, putting it to his head and dry-firing it, pretending to be Martin Riggs, sitting there thinking about suicide with a replica gun in his hand.) Or was it something else? That police tape across the kicked-in door. Did he have the weapons to hand for protection? Had everything been coming to a head recently? Sitting there in bed, with this fake gun that he couldn't afford any fake bullets for, watching his breath misting up towards the ceiling, unable to turn on a light, or boil a kettle, or . . . oh Jesus.

Why hadn't I written him a cheque? Why didn't he ask me to write him one? Because they don't, do they. Pride. You take it for as

130

long as you can and then you reach for the Stanley knife, you tie the noose. And I was forgetting something else: I had made it very clear I was getting sick of his shit.

The year before, the summer of 2009, and I have been lending Gary money more and more regularly. A hundred quid here. A couple of hundred there. Then, one afternoon he texts me: *John, u know anyone whod buy my golf clubs?*' Something about it infuriates me. The way he wasn't just coming right out asking for the money. That it had to be dressed up in this subterfuge. That I was obviously meant to say, 'Oh no! Why are you selling your golf clubs, Gary?' With a coldness that is mystifying to me in hindsight, I text back to say that he should just put them in the local paper, in the classified ads. He says he doesn't have enough money for the advert. Then he rings and tells me that he really does urgently need to borrow some money. A thousand pounds. He begins the story . . .

He'd been looking after a consignment of amphetamine sulphate for a bigger drug dealer. He hadn't wanted to keep it in the house so he'd buried it up in the woods but then he—

'Gary, can I stop you there?' I say. 'We've been here before . . .'

When he was released from prison, back in 1999, I'd told Gary that if he ever needed any help getting back on his feet then he only had to ask. I was in the living room of my flat in Maida Vale, west London, when the phone rang. It was Gary. He needed to borrow three thousand pounds because he'd agreed to look after a load of speed for some bigger dealer. Suddenly paranoid about having such a huge quantity of a class B drug in his house, especially as this would no longer be a first offence, he decided to bury the drugs in the

131

local woods. A simple 'X' marks the spot-type map would ensure their recovery. Gary promptly lost the map. The consignment of amphetamines was now forever hidden beneath the floor of Eglinton woods. Mr Big wasn't happy and for Gary it was now 'your money or your life' time.

'Eh?' I said, back in 1999.

'Aye, John. It'll be the wee thing wi' the silencer that goes *pfffft*.' He did the soft whisper of a silenced pistol.

'Come on,' I said. 'No one gets killed for three grand.'

And Shades sighed, 'Oh, John . . .' as he chuckled at my ivory-towered naivety, about my lack of understanding as to how the world really worked. The argument escalated, probably something to do with my reluctance to take his ludicrous story at face value, but, whatever the reason, Gary began screaming and shouting at me and I hung up. He rang back and, in his roughest, hardest whisper, hissed, 'You listen tae me, ya fucken prick, ye, if you ever hang up the phone on me again Ah'll come doon there tae London and Ah'll cut your throat.'

Gangster talk. Prison talk.

'You're aware that offering to cut my throat is an odd way to go about asking to borrow money?' I said.

Anyway, I gave him the three grand. And now here he was, ten years later, in 2009, telling me the exact same thing had happened again.

'Whit dae ye mean, "we've been here before"?' he asks.

'You already told me this exact story, Gary, ten years ago, when I lent you money.' I go through the whole thing. There is silence on the other end of the line. 'Now,' I go on in barrister-summing-up fashion, 'you're either so addled that you've completely forgotten about all that, or you're banking that I've forgotten about it, *or* you're genuinely asking me to believe that after the whole burying-drugs-in-the-woods thing worked out so well the last time, you decided to have another go. Seriously, which one of these guys do you want to be?'

A long pause before Shades says, 'I don't remember that.'

On the drive back to the hospital, Linda and I detour via the big, new police station on Kilwinning Road. I give the desk sergeant my brother's name and address and explain what has happened to him. Can he tell us why there was police tape across his front door? What had happened recently? He goes off and comes back a moment later with a plain clothes officer who takes me to one side and tells me softly that, yes, there was a police raid on my brother's house two days ago, but he can't give us any more information than that. 'All I can tell you, Mr Niven, is that your brother is, ah, "known to the police".' His inverted commas are almost audible.

'Surely,' I say, 'if he dies, then you can tell me more?'

'Not even then,' he says.

I call my university friend Donald, a criminal lawyer in Glasgow now, and ask him why – even if Gary is dead – the police still wouldn't be able to tell us anything about their dealings with him. 'The most likely reason,' Donald says, 'is because it might prejudice an open investigation. Something involving other people. It could compromise ongoing intelligence gathering.' The woods, the lost maps, the gun, the sword, hiding stuff for Mr Big. The wee thing with the silencer that goes *pfffft*. I tell him about the cannabis cupboard, describing the space. 'It's unlikely they'd have raided his house for, what, six or ten plants? But sometimes, if you've got enemies, they'll grass you in to try and

133

curry favour, or just because they don't like you, they'll tell the polis that you've got an actual factory on the go when you're just growing some for your own use. Then they follow up the lead, kick the door in, and end up with bugger all. But that's not to say, depending on what else you had going on, your previous, that you might not still end up in court . . .'

We get back to the hospital to find mum hasn't moved from Gary's bedside. 'Where have you two been?' she asks, agitated. 'The consultant wants to see us.'

We sit down with him in a small room provided for 'family consultations' – dusty plastic flowers on the table, pastel prints of soothing country scenes on the walls – and he tells us that, as we are now past the twenty-four-hour mark, they have gradually been withdrawing the drugs that have been keeping Gary in the coma.

'So,' mum says, hopeful as a child on Christmas morning, 'does that mean he'll wake up soon?'

'Unfortunately, if that was going to happen, I think it already would have,' the consultant says. 'The sedatives are pretty much out of his system now. I have to say that I think it's unlikely he'll regain consciousness at this point.'

'Have you done a CT scan yet?' I ask. 'Or an MRI?'

'No.'

'Can I ask why not?'

He looks at me. 'Well, Mr Niven, they wouldn't give us much more information than we already have. And they wouldn't help us with Gary's practical care at this point.' There is some more hackle-raising for me here, in the 'caring' way he uses my brother's name. It puts

134

me in mind of the many funerals I have been to, where the minister will casually, frequently, use the first name of someone they never met. I also have a quiet loop running in the back of my head now as I sit down with these people, one that gently but insistently repeats the words *'he hanged himself in your hospital'* over and over again. 'But,' he adds, 'I will be speaking to the director of clinical care about it.'

'Mmm,' I say, deciding it's not the best time to reveal I have a back channel to another consultant. 'Can I speak to them too, please?'

'I'll tell him you want to see him.'

A terseness is beginning to enter these exchanges.

'So what happens now?'

'Well, we'll continue to monitor him for the time being.'

You're still what? You're still collating?

Later that afternoon, mum finally asks me and Linda the question we've been waiting for – 'How long can he stay like this for?'

'Well, people have been in comas for weeks – months even – and recovered,' I say, parroting the most positive stories I've been reading online. As she brightens at this, I look at Linda. We need to tell her. It is past time to begin managing expectations. 'But a lot of it depends on how they wound up in the coma, mum. And the thing is . . . Gary's heart stopped for ten minutes, maybe longer. That's a long time for the brain to be deprived of oxygen. It means, even if he does wake up, there might be serious damage . . . to the brain.' It takes mum a couple of seconds to comprehend that the words 'brain' and 'damage' are being put together out loud in front of her for the first time. She starts to cry as Linda folds her into her arms, mum repeating the words 'Oh son, oh Gary, oh my God, oh son, oh my God' over and over.

135

Linda lives in Glasgow. I have been down south since the mid-90s. Mum and Gary have both remained here, in Ayrshire. In recent years, after he broke up with his fiancée, as his headaches worsened, as he gradually stopped working, mum has become Gary's sole caregiver. She has lent him money, a tenner here, twenty there. She has put together food packages for him, doing some extra shopping on top of her own and taking it up to his house. She's tried to help him manage the medication for his headaches. As neither Gary nor mum can drive, all of this has meant bus rides and a lot of walking for her. Since dad died and Linda and I moved away, mum and Gary have come to represent a distinct faction in the family. They are both Irvine people, with their *Daily Records*, their Mayfair cigarettes, their mince and tatties. They ride the same buses and walk the same streets and talk to each other about who they bumped into down the Cross. They have both lived and will both die in this town. They speak the same language, with their double positives, their 'so Ah dids' and their 'so it wizes'. And here's Linda and I – the Met Lib Elite, fannying about with our city lives, with our Nigella recipes and our Marlboro Lights. Mum is weeping not only for her son, but for her friend, her last remaining true ally in the family. The person who would take her side, someone with whom she can snort and chorus 'whit a load o' bloody rubbish!' when Linda or I start crapping on about something we've read in the *Guardian*. Or heard on Radio 4. Or BBC Two. (I once picked up the remote control from Uncle Drew's side table at Whyte Avenue back in the 90s to see that the buttons for channels 1 and 3 – BBC One and ITV – were almost worn out, illegible. The 2 and 4 buttons – BBC Two and Channel 4 – were pristine, literally untouched since the unit left the factory.) It dawns on me how much mum is going to miss Gary.

Because I'm already wondering about next steps. About insisting we perform a brain scan. Is it a money thing? Can we offer to pay privately? And then what? I'm already lurching towards what seems like the most awful outcome imaginable: Gary survives as a vegetable. He comes out of the coma having sustained the kind of massive brain damage that leaves him requiring twenty-four-hour, seven-days-a-week care for the rest of his life. There is only one possible candidate for this role. I picture mum, spooning the mush towards him. Turning him in his bed. Dressing him. Getting him into the wheelchair for a stroll down to the town. (*'Aye, he's fine. Just out for our wee walk, so we are. Come on then, Gary, son, better get ye back home before that rain comes.'*) Shades' staring, vacant eyes. The drool. And I know that, if he lives, she will do all of this, gladly. But it will mean the end of her life as she knows it, just as it has been starting to get back on a happier track with Eddie, more than fifteen years after dad died. I think about Fintan, sucking air in through his teeth and it dawns on me . . .

I am now very much hoping that my brother will die.

1983

'Happy Birthday, Danny'

As we both move further into our teens, Shades remains small for his age but continues to grow in fearlessness, and he begins to attain the kind of status small, fearless boys sometimes do with the older, bigger, harder kids, with the boys in the stonewash and the waffle jumpers: a kind of mascot. Not hard enough to be truly dangerous, but wild enough to be good value. The kid who will do anything. Throwing stones and shoes and shooting airguns begins to give way to more extreme transgressions. There's the extended burst of truancy. Then some shoplifting. An episode involving a complex scheme to embezzle video machines in the amusement arcade downtown, where he increasingly spends all his free time. All of this drives him and dad further and further apart. No more carpentry sessions in the garage. No more trips to the golf course. No more football in the back garden. In due course, Shades tries his hand at another zeitgeist tabloid favourite when, to celebrate his friend Danny's fifteenth birthday, they head over the moors with the crisp packets and the Evo-Stik. They get thoroughly spangled in some gorse bushes. At one point, Danny will tell me, years later, they are so high on glue that the two of them simultaneously hallucinate exactly the same thing: a light aircraft high above them, a plume of white smoke behind it as it skywrites the words 'HAPPY BIRTHDAY DANNY' in fifty-foot letters across the blue canopy.

Later, as they come staggering homewards along Kilwinning Road, a car pulls up beside them – Danny's dad. He tells them to hop in and they can drop Gary off on the way home. They look at each other – utterly bent on solvent – as they clamber onto the back seat and sit side by side, surreally off their nuts, the streets and houses outside morphing and melting as they turn onto Livingstone Terrace. They talk in hushed whispers, keeping their voices below the sound of Steve Wright in the afternoon purring from the radio as they debate the pros and cons of coming right out and asking Danny's dad if he'd really done it, if he had indeed hired a plane to skywrite 'Happy Birthday' across the skies of Ayrshire for his son. Wisely, they decide against this. Whether he's preoccupied, or has a poor sense of smell, or is simply incredibly unobservant, at no point does Danny's dad turn around to the back seat, at no point does he notice that his passengers are whacked out of their minds and reeking of glue.

Gary's return home is spectacular. He lurches through the front door – his legs skittering beneath him like a newborn colt, his eyes rainbow-pinwheeling in their sockets – to be greeted by me and, behind me, emerging from the kitchen, drying her hands on a dish-towel: mum. The front door is still open – I hear the cheerful parp of Danny and his dad driving off in the background – and then mum's cheery 'Hi, Gary, son!' is fast dying on her lips as she grabs Shades by the shoulders and takes him in.

He is *reeking* of glue.

Bits of crisp packet are stuck to his face.

Mum, who is very up on her tabloids, simply screams and then bursts into tears. Then she picks up the phone . . .

Danny had no idea that the fortunes of man could be so swiftly reversed in the space of a few minutes. They dropped Gary off and drove the half-mile to their own home, Danny in the back, enjoying the chauffeuring, enjoying his dad singing along to the radio as gently blurring pebbledash swirled past, one house after another, the millions of tiny stones, like Cadbury's Mini Eggs, as though some giant had thrown a shale beach across miles of wet cement. He walked into the house behind his father – his plan being to slope off to his room and quietly trip balls – only to see his mother standing in the hall, where the phone always lived in those days, the receiver still in her hand as her jaw dropped. In a movie our mum's voice would still have been coming out of that receiver as Danny's mum dropped it to her side, tears coming to her eyes as she pointed a trembling finger at her son and screamed the dread words . . .

'HE'S BEEN BUZZIN' THE GLUE WI' GARY NIVEN!'

And then Danny is crumpling beneath his father's beating with a single thought going through his mind as the fists descended: *fuck sake, Shades.*

Gary will suffer this too, later on, when dad gets home and his fists descend. But, the way Gary saw it at that point, everyone takes a beating now and then.

White Leather Biker's Jacket

I remedy the disgraceful, patchworked biker's jacket situation a year after I buy it, on my very first trip to London, a week after my seventeenth birthday in May 1983, when we all travel down by coach with Irvine Youth CND, to join 30,000 others at the GLC-sponsored 'Concert for Peace' in Brockwell Park, Brixton. As the 80s have unfolded, our friendship group has expanded. As well as the members of our bands there's now Larry Rhodes and Peter Padden and Haysee and Rab and Kevin McMunigal and now no less than three Andys: Kerr, Crone and O'Hagan, the last a couple of years younger than us and an interloper from Kilwinning, who writes a fanzine. We do the things you do: we put on gigs in the backrooms of pubs and stick posters up with wallpaper paste and rehearse in tiny bedrooms, the air thick with smoke and the tang of lager.

Basil is on the trip to London too. The former Sergeant Pieroni has become my new best friend and the manager of our band. Three years older than me, it is with Basil that I first begin exploring music that lies thrillingly, unthinkably, outside the strict parameters of punk rock. His family live in a small Orlit council house on Woodlands Avenue, opposite the old greyhound stadium, the dug track *('ye taking her up the dug track, aye?')*. It is in Basil's forever cold, mildly damp bedroom that he plays me Johnny Cash's *Live At Folsom Prison*, the Rolling Stones' *Some Girls* and Lou Reed's *Transformer*. In among his 7-inches he has the first three New Order singles and we even go as far as enjoying *Sultans Of Swing* by Dire Straits, although we definitely don't talk about that one beyond these four cold, damp walls. Here it was then, the older brother I never had. And the boundaries of music are not the only thing getting pushed at Woodlands Avenue. Basil's parents are second-generation Italian immigrants, which means an entrée to a whole other world I never knew about: food. There is always a deep pot of minestrone on the hob and fresh butter on the table. His mum will fry thick slabs of polenta studded with carrot,

144

celery, potato and tiny bits of bacon in a heavy-bottomed cast-iron pan until it is crisp and golden on the outside, soft and gooey on the inside. It all feels very far from our house around the corner, with our Findus Crispy Pancakes, our mince and tatties, our margarine, Potato Waffles and frozen French Bread Pizzas. Basil teaches me about food and music and, quid pro quo, I teach him his first few chords, on the massive, cheap, almost impossible to play Hondo acoustic guitar he's bought.

After the concert in Brockwell Park, we have the evening to kill before the midnight coach back to Glasgow. Being provincial teenagers, we head for the only place in London we've ever heard of – Carnaby Street. As soon as I see it in the window of the shop I know I must have it. It is snow-white, its shell smooth and creamy and untouched by any humiliating patchwork stitching. Its lining of satin is as red as the revolution. It screams 'rock star'. My pockets are swollen with ill-gotten milk-round cash and I fork out an incredible seventy pounds to buy it on the spot: the White Leather Biker's Jacket.

With me unable to fully move my arms in my new casing, smelling like a fresh three-piece suite and walking with the stiff, rotating-from-the-waist motion of C3PO, we set off, our footsteps taking us further south, into a place called Soho, which looks familiar from TV, from photos of the early days of punk. People from pubs spill out onto the pavement, drinking in the warm dusk. There are coloured bulbs strung along the market stalls, bright neon starting to come on now too: 'RAYMOND'S REVUE BAR', signs with black lettering on yellow saying 'PEEP SHOW' and 'BLUE FILMS'. Strange door-ways advertising 'MODELS'. It is all madly intoxicating. With Basil taking point, we gain entry to a big boozer on Cambridge Circus called the Spice of Life. As we jostle near the crowded Saturday evening bar one of us says 'fucking hell . . .' and we all turn to look.

There's a bunch of guys with quiffs and denim and leather jackets, smoking up a storm at a corner table littered with glasses. Our jaws start to drop as we realise that a couple of them look familiar. Very familiar. Which they should do.

It's The Clash.

Well, half of The Clash to be precise. Once again, it's the duo of Strummer and my old pal Paul Simonon, surrounded by a load of mates. Yes, we have come to a city of eight million people and have somehow chosen to drink in the very same pub as The fucking Clash. Even at a distance of some yards, and with the crush of many bodies between us, I am breaking out in a light sweat from the proximity rush. Basil and I look at each other: this can't actually be happening.

We order pints and lurk as close to their group as we can without looking like mental stalkers begging to get thrown out. One of the guys in the entourage is Kosmo Vinyl, who less than a year earlier cut Basil's hair into a Mohawk backstage at the Magnum Centre. Would this form the basis for an introduction, we wonder? But we're just too scared. We drink and talk in low voices, speculating once again about why Mick isn't with them. What we did not, could not know, that night in the Spice of Life on Cambridge Circus, with our pints still like huge German steins in our teenage fists, is that in two weeks' time The Clash will fly to America, to begin a string of warm-up dates before their appearance at the US Festival in California: it will be the last time Mick Jones ever sets foot onstage with the band. What we do not know, as we stand there gawking is, that in May 1983

Strummer and Simonon are just three months away from firing the guitarist they have come to hate with a near-biblical passion. As the lagers slide down, I gain confidence. Probably best to avoid Paul, given, you know. But eventually I spot Strummer making his way through the crowd, heading towards the toilets. *This is it.*

After a few seconds I head through the crush. On my way towards the door marked 'GENTS', the door that just closed behind Strummer, I have time to wonder about tactics. What if he's having a crap? Slide a note under? Begin conversation through the door? Loiter until he emerges and open with a cheery 'Good shite, Joe?' Thankfully, as I come through the door, Strummer is at the urinal, and he's the only other person in the tiny, tiled Victorian toilet. He stands with his back to me at the trough, the reek of an afternoon of London drinking sour in the air. I take my place at the other end of the porcelain bower – the notion of Joe Strummer acciden-tally thinking I might be trying to look at his penis unthinkable to me – and stare straight ahead, my cheeks reddening, my mind crum-bling as I try to come up with an opener. Obviously, a further complication is that I can no more make water than conversation: the only sound is that of the steady, blissful stream being generated by one of the greatest frontmen of his generation, the man who changed our lives.

It is, I reflect, quite a journey I have been on these past four years, from seeing his face for the first time on the poster in Craig Russell's bedroom to here, in Soho, listening to the powerful drill of his urine, just feet away from me. Finally, Strummer finishes and zips up. He starts washing his hands. *Think.* Suddenly I have it. A foolproof opener. Casual and conversational. Not too fanboy, but less confrontational than my Simonon gambit last summer. It is an opener that shows I am no casual fan, but not too trainspotterish either. I absolutely cannot go wrong with this one.

'Hey, Joe,' I say cheerfully. Strummer, drying his hands on a paper towel, allows a small, tolerant smile. I am, after all, a seventeen-year-old boy with a bad quiff in a leather jacket. He knows the kind of thing that's coming. 'Where's Mick?'

Strummer's face instantly darkens, his eyes narrowing. 'I don't fucking know!' he snarls, tossing the paper towel in the bin, turning on his heel and striding out the door.

It is some time before I leave the bathroom.

'What did he say? What did he say?' Basil asks.

'Ach, not much . . .'

Later, on the ten-hour coach trip back to Glasgow, I ruminate on the fact that, if I only knew where Mick Jones lived, then I could complete the set by managing to offend every single original member of the band.

And there was more stuff I did not know as we headed north up the M6 in the early hours of that Sunday morning, on 8 May 1983. I did not know, as we passed the turn-off for the M56 towards Manchester, that the following week a band from that city would release their debut single. I did not know that by the time this band put out their second single that September, they would mean everything to me that The Clash had for the last three years. The faces of Strummer and Jones would fall from my wall.

INT. LIVING ROOM – DAY

A working-class space: electric 'coal-effect' fire etc.

A MAN (late 50s, greying hair, shirt and clip-on tie) and a BOY (16, semi-mullet, waffle jumper and slip-on shoes) are eating mince, tatties and beans in front of the TV, both stirring their food into a pink mush. This is DAD and GARY.

CHYRON ONSCREEN: 'IRVINE, AYRSHIRE. SUMMER 1984'

Dad is channel hopping when a THIRD FIGURE enters. He's wearing a plum blouse from Evans outsize women's wear, with the collar cut off, a chain of red plastic beads around his neck, faded jeans and Hush Puppies. His hair is teased into an amateur approximation of Morrissey's quiff. This is JOHN (18).

> JOHN
> Good evening, Pater. Brother.

They grunt. John peers incredulously at their plates.

> JOHN
> And what is the bill of fare tonight, pray tell? The trout Almondine? Steak tartare?

> DAD
> Mince and tatties.

                    JOHN
        Goodness! How retro!

                    GARY
        You ur such a bentshot, pal.

                    JOHN
        Tell me, how will we be spending this
        Saturday evening? If I may . . .

He theatrically produces a copy of the *NME*,
consults it.

                    JOHN
        I see the new Wim Wenders film *Paris,*
        Texas is on nationwide release.
        Perhaps we could catch it at the GFT?
        Or there's the 'terrifying' nuclear
        war drama *Threads* on BBC Two later
        tonight. No?

They both continue to ignore him. Dad suddenly
thumbs the volume up on the remote. A familiar
theme tune blares out . . .

                    TV
        'In 1972, a crack commando unit was
        sent to prison by a military court
        for a crime they didn't commit . . .'

Dad and Gary both lock into THE A TEAM, transfixed.

                    150

                    JOHN
Or there's that . . .
                    (beat)
Closer to home, I couldn't interest
you in local Joy Division copyists
Dead Souls live at the Grange Hotel?

                    GARY
Gaunnae shut it, ya bender?

                    DAD
Aye, gies peace, John.

                    JOHN
Very well. I shall away!

Wings

Gary leaves Ravenspark in the summer of 1984, aged sixteen, with no qualifications, and starts signing on, his drifting, aimless existence fuelling the tensions in the house I was about to leave. Driven by bin-man terror, I'd 'stuck in' at 'the school', getting four Highers: a C, two Bs and a single A in English. Which makes my parents very proud. But . . . I talk funny, a little like Dolores Haze to her doomed mother, with my mannerisms and my big words and my judgements. Standing there in my daft clothes, with my daft haircut, I crap on about strange books and records and films. In many ways, on the dole or not, Gary is entirely more understandable to them. Sometimes dad would muse that perhaps the stork had 'dropped you down the wrong bloody chimney, John'. On the walls of my tiny bedroom upstairs, the faces of Roddy Frame and Edwyn Collins joined those of Morrissey and Marr. And it wouldn't be mine for much longer . . .

I arrive in Hillhead, in the West End, in the first week of October 1984, to read English Literature at Glasgow University. My parents drop me off at the flat on Gibson Street and, after we've unloaded the bin bags of clothes and the stereo, my few books and records, dad looks sheepish while mum cries in the street as she says her goodbyes. She hands me a parting gift, a tea towel bearing the legend –

The first thing we give our children is roots.
The last is wings.

I would give a great deal to still have that tea towel in my possession today. But sadly, its terrible destiny was to be press-ganged into taking over the horror-tasks of the 1978 Scotland World Cup top.

The first thing I put up on the wall of my shared bedroom is a picture of Morrissey I've cut out of the *NME*. However, by 1985, The Smiths are firmly established in the Imperial Phase of their career, meaning that anyone shallow and craven enough to want to be thought hip and happening (and, boy, am I shallow and craven) is having to nose out new bands to become obsessed with. It's the dawn of 'shambling', of what will come to be called 'indie': alabaster boys in stripy Breton tops, consumptive girls in woolly tights. To evoke those times, you perhaps need only a list: The Soup Dragons, The Chesterfields, One Thousand Violins, Close Lobsters, The Bodines, The Mighty Lemon Drops, Meat Whiplash, BMX Bandits, The Submarines, The Clouds, The June Brides.

We see most of these groups at Splash One, on West George Street, but our favourites are The Loft, who have even been on TV, performing their indie mega-smash 'Up The Hill And Down The Slope' on the *Oxford Road Show*. Then they split acrimoniously onstage in 1985, with lead singer Pete Astor going on to form The Weather Prophets

153

and bass player Bill Prince forming The Wishing Stones, for whom he becomes singer, guitarist and songwriter.

Having finally learned to play the guitar properly, my 80s have passed in a series of bad teenage bands with terrible two-word names – Suspect Device, Rebel Dance, Almost Evening, Celebrate Texas – who played first in my hometown, then further afield in Ayrshire – in Kilmarnock and Ayr – and then, finally, at the end of my teens, in Glasgow. In 1986, my band supports The Wishing Stones at Lucifer's, a basement club on Jamaica Street. Fifty indie kids frowning through their fringes, motionless, clutching pints. In the way of the times, no one has money for hotels and we put them up at our flat. Bill and I hit it off, sharing similar tastes in guitars, boots and New York bands of the mid-70s. We take them around Glasgow, to Paddy's Market, the Griffin bar, the Grosvenor café, the King's café, where Bill watches in horror as the slice of pizza he's ordered as a safeguard against anything too deep-fried is duly dropped into the deep-fat fryer.

We agree to stay in touch.

Ned Walk

A Saturday night in 1986. I'm back home from Glasgow for the weekend, ironing a shirt in the walk-through room that once belonged to Linda, who is now thirteen and in my old bedroom, just through the partition wall. After mum briefly experimented with using the walk-through as a kind of upstairs dining room, it has now become a kind of small lounge.

My enchantment with all things Creation Records has reached such a pitch that it has motivated the purchase of the leather trousers I am

154

now wearing as I iron. I had been in this very room a few weeks earlier – drinking cans with all the boys as we prepared to head out for the night – when dad burst dramatically through the door. Wearing his string vest, the lower half of him stuffed into my leather trousers, he cries, 'HO, BOYS! AM A NO DEAD WITH IT?' His fists on his hips, as he jutted his bum provocatively towards my friends. The outrage of his mad cheeks, a couple of footballs crammed into black pudding casing, the vest and the leather making him look like some ancient refugee from the Meatpacking District circa 1978.

'Jesus, dad,' I muttered beneath the gale of laughter from my pals. But I have learned to take these slings and arrows from my embarrassingly provincial family, who could not name you a single member of The Weather Prophets between them.

Shades, eighteen now, is still living at home, up in the attic room that has become his private domain. By the mid-80s he's become a proper wee ned, with a burgeoning reputation. On one of her first days at Ravenspark, Linda found herself cornered in the toilets by a trio of older, harder girls. She shrank back, waiting for the demand for her lunch money, for whatever. Then one of them saw her name on the jotters she clutched to her chest.

'Linda *Niven*?'

'Aye.'

'Oh tae fuck. Are you . . . Shades' wee sister?'

'Aye.'

'Yer aw right, hen. Nae bother. Come on, youse . . .'

And the three of them back away, giving her assurances as they do so that not only would they never attempt to mess with her again, it was pretty certain that no one would. She was, she felt, *protected*.

Shortly after I leave home, Shades also attempts to do so. No UCCA forms, flat-hunting or government grants are involved in the process. Around his seventeenth birthday, an argument with dad over his jobless, directionless life climaxed with Shades telling dad to fuck off, storming out of the house and going to live with his mate in a tent in the woods behind Eglinton country park. Linda witnessed his departure: the screaming row on the doorstep, the rucksack over his back, mum crying and trying to hold him back, Shades screaming, 'GET AFF ME! LEE ME ALANE!'

Being thirty miles away and wrapped up in my own life – Queequeg's harpoon, Milton's blindness, *Rattlesnakes* by Lloyd Cole and the Commotions, Fürstenberg beer – I don't remember thinking too much about this episode at the time. Looking back now it seems improbably surreal: Shades as Huck Finn, or Hemingway's Nick Adams, cooking tinned beans on a camping stove, chopping down branches for his fire, casting a line into a brook to chance for trout. Or, perhaps more accurately, Shades as *Jerusalem*'s Rooster Byron: lager and sulphate and ranting. Although these notions are undercut by the fact that, during the few summer weeks of 1985 he spent in this bucolic idyll, he would routinely pop back with washing for mum to do. A peace was eventually brokered with dad that allowed Shades to return home and, soon after, he finally found a job, on the shop floor at Fullarton Fabrications, at the time the biggest employer in Irvine, with five factories and a workforce of nearly a thousand. He is now earning a wage from honest toil. He is working a lathe and will routinely remind you that he has 'hands like leather'. He'll flash his wad in your student face in true 'loadsamoney' style as he gets a round in while you sit there, counting your change.

I'm ironing when I hear the clank of Shades' feet coming down

the aluminium stepladder from his loft bedroom, and then he's sauntering into the room in the strutting ned walk he's refining: a kind
of shoulder-jutting pimp stroll. He opens with a solid volley . . .

'Whit ye daeing, ya massive bender?'

'What does it look like, ya wee dick?'

He smirks as he takes in the paisley shirt on the ironing board, the
leather trousers. Shades is in his uniform too: leisurewear, a baggy
sweatshirt with a thin gold chain around his neck. There's a smouldering Kensitas Club in his fist and two chunky gold rings glinting
on his fingers. 'Whit,' he says slowly, shaking his head, despairing, 'kind
o' a fucking shirt dae ye call that?'

'Piss off.'

He snatches the shirt off the ironing board, holds it up against
himself and starts mincing and simpering about, his voice going up
an octave as he coos . . .

'Ohh, Ah'm Morrissey so Ah um. Ah'm bent. Oooohhh, take me up the
erse, big boy. Ride me daft.'

'Gimme it back, you clown.'

'Ur you bent, John?' he asks, getting right in my face, asking it with
maximum urgency, as though his very life depends upon my answer.
'Ur you actually bent, ya mad hom, ye?'

I snatch the shirt back and go to bat him around the head, to swat
him away like a fly, as I've done countless times since childhood. He
grabs my hand before it reaches him and quickly twists it around my
back, his grip amazingly strong, his reflexes fast, as he drives my arm
painfully up towards my shoulder blades. His face comes close to mine,
grinning, leering. Then he shoves me away, patting my cheek playfully.
'See ye later, wee sacks.'

As he pimp strolls out, whistling, it dawns on me that, like so many other parts of childhood – like catching frogs, Chron Gen singles and Birds Eye Potato Waffles – shoving Shades around was now definitely a thing of the past.

Writing #1

In my first year at university, late at night, alone in the flat, I begin doing the same terrible, sordid thing that millions of English Literature undergraduates have done before me: I attempt short stories.

I send one into a competition in the student newspaper, the *Glasgow Guardian*, where I land my first-ever review, one I can still quote verbatim for you today – *'There was wit too, and a certain originality, in John Niven's "Of His Surgery and Beyond", but Mr Niven seemed confused as to the perspective from which to tell his story.'* My 3,000-worder was about a golfer, a dentist, who kills a girl with an errant drive that sails through the window of a nearby library. I can still recall the first sentence – 'The ball left the tee with a clean, clear snap' – and a single metaphor – 'his golf slacks and polo shirt betrayed him as effectively as a hangman's hood', and I recall being particularly pleased with that title. A few years later, my cheeks will flush with shame when I'm reading Martin Amis's review of Norman Mailer's sub-par 1980 novel *Of Women and Their Elegance* and find him saying, *'the "Of" of the title almost guaranteeing the vulgarity of the whole enterprise'*. Oof.

Safe to say I had very little in the way of talent or taste back then, and even less self-discipline. But I'd loved the process, sitting at the battered green Olivetti I'd picked up in the charity shop on Byres Road and pounding the story out. I liked the way the pages of typescript stacked up beside you, and I got an early intimation of the mathematics of writing, of the difficulties of structure, of the troubling fact that cranking out snappy dialogue is by far the least of your troubles. Of course, I had no way of knowing it back then, in the shared bedroom in the flat on Gibson Street, but very little is ever truly wasted for a writer. It just takes a while: twenty years later, I would circle back to the idea of someone being hit on the head by a stray golf ball for the plot kicker of *The Amateurs*.

So, I liked the idea of the writing life very much, yes, but at the age of twenty I was still too much in thrall to another kind of imagined life, the kind that involved amplifiers, guitars and the back of Transit vans.

Train Heaves on to Euston

April 1987. We're drinking in the Griffin, playing at spotting members of Primal Scream or The Pastels among the wooden, glass-panelled booths when, as in a film, the barman appears at the end of the bar, phone clutched to his chest as he shouts out, 'John Niven? Is there a John Niven in here?' My first thought is that it's a wind-up. The second, someone's died. But no, it's Bill Prince, calling from London. Knowing that we have no phone in our student flat we've kept in touch by letter and postcard, and saw each other for a few days the previous winter, he's gambled that we might be drinking in here. Pressing a finger into my ear, leaning on the wet mahogany, I listen as Bill tells me that he's sacked the Wishing Stones guitarist and would I be willing to step in and play guitar on an eleven-date UK tour supporting The Wedding Present? The first gig is less than two weeks away, so I'd have to come to London as soon as possible to start rehearsals. They'll pay my expenses and send train tickets and I can stay with Bill and his girlfriend Stephanie in Leytonstone. It'll involve taking some time out of university, of course. What do I think?

I think that Bill has been in the *NME* many times. He *writes* for the *NME*. The Wishing Stones have already released two singles on Head Records, also home to The Servants and a new band called Loop. It's run by a guy called Jeff Barrett, who also does press for Creation. I think that Bill was in The Loft, *giants* in our world, a world where indie music is still a quiet pond, not connected to the mainstream by any sort of tributary, where bands are largely unbothered by major record labels, where you could receive a full-page review in the music press, or pack out clubs and still remain unmolested by a single phone call from an A&R man. This is before that sort of thing really happened. Pre-Oasis. Pre-Stone Roses. In our world of underachievement and microscopic ambition, The Wishing Stones might as well be the Rolling Stones. What do I think? I think I'm Ronnie Wood, and I feel much as he must have done as he surveyed the itinerary for his first tour with the Stones back in 1975.

I turn twenty-one at midnight on 30 April in the back of a Transit van, wedged in amongst the amplifiers and guitar cases, with cans of lager being passed around and Mott The Hoople blaring. I have a Fender Telecaster and a Vox AC30. We have a driver/tour manager. There are backstage passes and itineraries and free beer and the stages are not made of milk crates, except for once, possibly, at Hull Adelphi. I am living my own personal teenage dream. It is the first time I have ever travelled around England, the first time I have seen

160

the huge blocks of bright yellow we pass on the springtime country roads: fields of rapeseed, like giant slabs of butter fallen from the sky.

I get to know the touring landmarks of Great Britain, names evocative of that time even now – Scotch Corner, Charnock Richard, Newport Pagnell, Watford Gap, Keele – as we make our way around the UK, staying in bed and breakfasts, or on the floors of friends or fans, gobbling Sudafed to stay awake and sipping Night Nurse to come down. Occasionally, there will be a match head of dope or a gram of speed. Our partial namesakes circa 1975 have nothing to fear. It's late at night and we're driving back to London after the last date on The Wedding Present tour, in Canterbury. Kent slides by in the dark, then the M2. Medway Services. I'm sitting up front, speeding and drinking lager with Jeff Barrett who runs our record label, Head.

'Thanks for doing the tour, John,' he says. 'Really saved the day, mate.'

'My pleasure. Been great.'

Jeff lights a Marlboro Red, his Zippo flashing in the dark. 'Now we've just got to find a way to keep you down here, haven't we?'

Shades is incredulous. 'Yer moving tae London? Fucking *London*?' As Shades sees it, moving to London in the autumn of 1987 can only mean one thing. 'Ye gaunnae get that AIDS pumped up ye, aye?'

'They don't hand out syringes of it on the train once you pass Carlisle, Gary.'

'Aye, it'll no be a syringe fur you. It'll–'

'Yeah, it'll be–'

161

'It'll be a coack.'

'Yes, I get it.'

'A big, black coack right up ye, John.'

Incredibly, mum and dad are far more understanding than my brother when I tell them I'm dropping out of university and moving four hundred miles away for reasons not much better than 'what can a poor boy do, 'cept to play for a rock and roll band?' The conversation takes place late at night in their bed, the locus of many a heart-to-heart during my teenage years. I sit on the bottom of the bed, drunk on Holsten Pils and possibility, while I tell them what I am going to do. Dad smokes, half watching the portable TV over my shoulder. The white MFI bedside cabinets, their matching ashtrays in dark, dimpled purple glass, my parents being of the last generation to smoke in bed. I tell them I can always return to my studies in the unlikely event that we're not headlining stadiums within the year. Dad tuts a bit and shakes his head and asks if I'm sure I know what the bloody hell I'm doing. Mum frets about 'that London', but basically they trust in the Hollywood truism of 'following your dreams'. It is in some ways a blessing that I am the first generation of my family to have gone to university – nothing is expected.

Shades continues to be less encouraging. 'Ach, it'll be a load o' pish,' he says. 'Like aw that shite you like.'

'What shite?'

'Aw that' – he mimes strumming a guitar while doing the whining croak of his 'indie' voice – '*aww, Ah'm dyin'* shite.' I patiently explain to my stupid, uncool brother about how the *NME* loved the last Wishing Stones single. About how Bill was in The Loft, about how we're going on tour with the–

'John,' Shades interrupts. 'Nobody cares about aw your pish. They're no even *paying* you, fur fuck sake.'

On this last point, he is undoubtedly correct. I'll be signing on. But, like many a fool before me, I figure, 'Hey, at least you'll get to hear the band play.' I also figure it's only going to take a couple of years before we're headlining Dingwalls. Maybe somewhere even bigger. Before the major record companies come calling with huge advances and promises of worldwide tours.

For 1988 was sure to be the year the UK finally came around to the allure of pale boys in polka-dot shirts playing a cross-breed of New York rock circa 1975 and The Band, wasn't it? A year, two tops, I tell mum and dad, and we'll be in the charts.

'Twenty quid *each?*'

I move to London on Sunday, 18 October: just two days after the Great Storm of 1987 has ripped through England. The Leytonstone we arrive in has trees torn from pavements and strewn across roads, the windows of cars and houses smashed by flying roof tiles. I take all of this as a good omen: the hurricane announcing, prefiguring, the drama of my arrival in the capital. We get our pictures in the *NME*, *Sounds* and *Melody Maker*, a big one in the *NME* too, with me scrubbing at my Telecaster onstage in Camden. It accompanies a five-star, half-page review by the paper's then editor Danny Kelly. We tour the UK several times, supported by label mates Loop, by Lush, by The Telescopes and by a few utterly hopeless new groups like the Milltown Brothers and Claytown Troupe. We record our debut album at Greenhouse Studios in Shoreditch, where Primal

Scream, The Wonder Stuff and The House of Love have all been recording their debut albums. But, as 1988 unfolds . . .

Outside London, it's a good gig if we walk onstage to an audience of more than fifty people. Many nights there are just a handful of indie kids scattered around, clinging to the walls. And, unlike all those other Greenhouse groups, no major labels are coming a-calling. In fact, opening for The Wishing Stones becomes a guaranteed ticket to indie stardom: Loop handily leapfrog us and are soon headlining ULU. Likewise Lush, who soon sign to 4AD. The Telescopes sign to Creation and the Milltown Brothers to A&M. In final-insult territory, even the bastard Claytown Troupe get signed to Island for big money, a fact dismally confirmed when they support us for a second time and we notice the price tags still stuck on their gleaming stacks of brand-new Marshalls. By the summer we are so poor that our bass player The Bull and I are grateful when Barrett pays us each thirty quid and a few pints of Guinness to spend an afternoon slapping black paint on the walls of the backroom of a Camden pub called the Falcon, where he's moving his gigs from the Black Horse. And there's other complicated stuff in the air, that summer . . .

I have begun an affair with – and fallen in love with – Bill's girlfriend Stephanie. Steph is four years older than me, beautiful and worldly, and obviously tensions begin to run high when Bill learns of the situation. Had the band been becoming more successful we might have got past all of this somehow: it's likely easier to ride out love triangles when you're the Rolling Stones circa 1968, on the private jet on the way to Oakland Coliseum. In The Wishing Stones in 1988, in the Transit van on the way to Northampton Roadmenders, it's more difficult. The tension between Bill and me, the tiny audiences, the poverty in a time and place as indifferent to it as the London of the late 80s (the newsreel footage here: stockbrokers in red braces spraying champagne, Thatcher, Porsches, graphs going up-up-up), it all gradually starts to become overwhelming. There's also the fact that pale boys in Chelsea boots with guitars are beginning to look like Penny Farthings, like cave paintings, like dad's beloved Herb Albert albums.

That August, on a hot night, a few of us go to a friend's birthday party at their house over in Walthamstow, where we're looking forward to the usual kind of time had by indie musicians of the time – lager and a few joints. Maybe whisky and some speed if things really get out of hand. The evening takes an unexpected turn when a friend-of-our-friend brings out a small tin and opens it to reveal lots of little white pills – it is this so-called 'ecstasy' the tabloids have been banging on about. We're keen, but, cool your boots, man, because . . .

'They're twenty quid.'

'For how many?'

'Twenty quid *each*,' the man says.

'*What?* Jesus. Can you take half of one?'

The good doctor shakes his head.

This is a *staggering* amount of cash. Our dole money is thirty pounds a week, plus the odd hundred and fifty between the four of us for a gig, plus the stray income from whatever venue-painting Jeff might need done. After a hurried conference, three of us pool our resources and are just about able to scrape together sixty pounds between us to cover a pill per man.

We wash them down with Red Stripe and resume politely discussing the burning issues of the day in our world: the overproduction of the new Go-Betweens album, *16 Lovers Lane*. Can we get on the guest list for Felt at ULU next week? Why are Primal Scream taking so long to record the follow-up to *Sonic Flower Groove*?

Fast-forward an hour.

We're all in a scrum on the floor, glowing, vibrating, filled with a fathomless love for every single creature on earth as we collectively come up on a rush that feels like being strapped to the front of a locomotive. We're listening to Iggy Pop's 1977 live album *TV Eye* and – *HOLY SHIT, I've never thought about it before, but this is LITERALLY the greatest music ever recorded.* And how incredible would it be to be hearing this music surrounded by hundreds, thousands, of people on the same drug? All experiencing it at the same time in exactly the same way? And who knows, and difficult as it is to imagine it right now – as I crawl towards the bathroom for what will be the most pleasurable bout of vomiting I have ever experienced – but perhaps there was even better music to listen to on ecstasy than Iggy Pop live? Because, although none of us quite know it yet, as we lie on our backs listening to Iggy scream, watching the ceiling pulse and throb like a womb, across town a club called Shoom has recently moved from a tiny venue in Southwark to a much larger one on Tottenham Court Road. What we are experiencing is nothing less than the gathering rush of our own musical doom.

Four hundred miles north, someone is already answering the questions I'm asking myself on that bathroom floor in Walthamstow. Rave hits Scotland hard over the summer of 1988. While I'm still wondering why The Weather Prophets aren't having more chart success, or discussing the merits of the Vox AC30 versus the Fender Twin Reverb, or whatever the fuck, those little white pills are snowing down over Glasgow. Slam begin their club nights at Tin Pan Alley in the city centre. Soon enough they're hosting packed all-nighters at the Tramway Theatre on the Southside: 808 State, Derrick May, Rebel MC and Kevin Saunderson. It starts trickling out into the provinces, down into Ayrshire. Streetrave start their parties at Ayr Pavilion, where, a lifetime ago, I watched The UK Subs. Soon Ayr Pavilion isn't big enough and they're throwing parties in Prestwick Airport, at ice rinks, in arenas. Rave nights launch at the Metro in Saltcoats, and even in Irvine, at the Pleasuredome, above the Co-op.

Shades hasn't had much truck with music through his late teens, but the combination of ecstasy and this new, pummelling immersive soundtrack seduces him utterly. I only get fragments from mum's letters to London: *'Gary's moved into a wee flat with his pals . . . probably for the best . . . him and dad were arguing a lot . . . he's doing fine . . . having a good time . . .'*

Shoulder-Rolling Pimp Stroll

A freezing cold winter's night in January 1989, I'm in bed at our rented house in Leytonstone, watching *The Other Side of Midnight* on my little black-and-white portable TV. The late-night chat and music show is hosted by Factory Records boss Tony Wilson, who looks into the camera and says, 'Now, a Manchester group whose rock and roll stance I have seriously disliked for four or five years . . . here's the new one from the excellent Stone Roses . . .'

Now, I'd heard of this band, but I hadn't paid too much attention to them. You always saw posters for their shows all over town whenever you played in Manchester. I'd heard their last single, 'Elephant-something' a few times. It was all right. A swirling, chiming riff comes out of the tiny TV speaker as the camera cuts to four guys on the plain white stage. The guitarist is playing a big Gretsch and he's wearing what looks to be . . . leisure wear. A black and white baggy sweatshirt. The singer is in a polo shirt, with his hand briefly on his hip before he starts this kind of shoulder-rolling stroll as the tune unfolds, the groove sophisticated, the rhythm section locked together, the bassline fluid and loping, the drummer in constant motion, wearing a weird kind of hat as he does most of the song on the hi-hat, with the occasional filigree around the kit. It's *almost* the kind of guitar music I've lived with for the last four or five years, but not. And forget *TV Eye*, imagine dancing to *this* on ecstasy. The singer increasingly makes direct eye contact with the camera, kind of defiant yet nervous at the same time, his eyes darting, almost guilty-looking, his pimp strut more emboldened as the song builds.

I'm sitting up in bed now, closer to the tiny TV, as he juts his way around in a way very familiar to me.

And there, gleaming under the studio lights on the fingers of Ian Brown's right hand as the camera moves in closer . . .

Two chunky gold rings.

Fucking Shades.

Who is, of course, way, way ahead of me.

The creeping suspicions of the last few months suddenly crystallise into an epiphany: we're The Tornadoes in the winter of 1962 hearing the confident stomp of 'Love Me Do' on the radio for the first time.

We're done.

Writing #2

There's been something else bubbling under too, towards the end of the band. At the kitchen table, pounding away on my old Olivetti, I've been trying to write a novel, a kind of detective story about a series of murders. I still have the pages, more than thirty years later, and it's embarrassing in all the ways a novel attempted by someone in their early twenties usually is: self-conscious, mannered and confused.

And it's insanely, graphically, violent – killings involving things like petrol enemas that turn 'insides to lasagne'. I give up after a hundred pages or so. I have no idea where I am going with it. It's just too hard. At twenty-two I lack the self-discipline required to shut the world out for two to five hours every single day for six months or a year. I lack the focus you need to get to the end, to type 'THE END' and then, incredible to me then, to turn back to page one and begin the monumental task of the second draft, where you will have to throw out huge chunks of what you have done. (Because I do not yet know the truism *writing is rewriting*.) I do not know that I won't have these qualities for more than a decade, until I am in my early thirties. Nabokov said that the idea of retiring to your ivory tower to write is all very well, but in order to build it, you must first take the unavoidable trouble of killing quite a few elephants. And here I was – elephantless. But trying to write the novel has started me reading them again, after all that time in the back of a Transit van, with the copies of *Viz* and the arguments over whether Mick Ralphs or Mick Ronson was the better guitar player. I find myself thinking about the English degree I walked out on two years earlier. Stephanie and I want to live together and she's saved the money towards a deposit on a flat. But London is going through its late-80s property boom, with a two-up-two-down in Walthamstow going for an incredible *eighty thousand pounds* (a hilarious joke there for readers under forty). Glasgow, however, is still much more reasonably priced. I call the university and find out that I am *just* in time to be readmitted in October, back into the third year of my course. Stephanie begins looking for a job in Glasgow and we buy a one-bedroom attic flat in the West End for thirty grand, taking out a mortgage at the then bargain interest rate of 15%. Our payments will be three hundred quid a month. We take on this terrible responsibility and I move back to Glasgow in August 1989, the week after fifty-one people drown in the Thames when a huge dredger hits a pleasure cruiser. In the end, like I told my parents, it did take less than two years. I'd arrived in a hurricane, in October 1987, and left in the wake of a disaster, the mini-tragedy of my personal failure overwhelmed by the fact that the twenty-two months I spent in London somehow managed to encompass the Great Storm, Black Monday, the King's Cross fire, the Clapham rail crash, Lockerbie, Hillsborough and the sinking of the *Marchioness*.

Just like the boy said – *no one cared about all our pish.*

Up the Pole

And here comes the boy himself, with a cheery *'Awright, wee sacks?'* Shades is already fully onboard, standing on the sharp prow of the future, in Stone Island and Armani jeans and Timberland boots. And there's me: in polka-dot shirt and Paddy's Market suit jacket, clinging to the old ways like a bewildered Ted during psychedelia. Armed with his now ever-present Rizlas, Shades skins up as he slips 'French Kiss' or 'Voodoo Ray' or 'Back To Life' on the turntable up in the attic at Livingstone Terrace, where he's moved back in. Rent difficulties.

A few weeks after I resume my course, I sit sipping a pint in the Griffin on a cold November night. The Glasgow I've returned to is very different from the one I left two years ago, let alone the one I first arrived in back in 1984. Back then Primal Scream had just played their first show across the road at the Venue, supporting the Mary Chain. Tonight, *Top of the Pops* is showing on the TV above the door: the Roses and the Mondays are both on. A few months later, the Primals themselves will be on the show too, resplendent in luminous rave colours as 'Loaded' swirls disconnected around them. While I've been in London, Lucifer's on Jamaica Street has become the Sub Club.

Symbolically, it's where my band supported The Wishing Stones just three short years ago, those three years now being the difference between 1964 and 1967, between a suit and tie and satin loon pants, between a pint of bitter and a blotter of acid, between 'Telstar' and 'Sunshine Of Your Love'. And the place is no longer half-filled with shy indie kids, motionless and clutching beers. The three-thousand-square-foot basement sweatbox is now *rammed* every weekend, with four hundred twentysomethings ripped to the gills on what Stuart and Orde are playing and those little white pills we had at that party.

It is here that Shades and much of my old crowd from Irvine now head on a weekend. There's Keith and Larry and all the Andys and – incredibly – they're all sitting in the corner with our cousins, with David and Kevin, and Shades and his mates. There's Vouchers and Sconzo and Tony and even Linda, now seventeen, in regulation dungarees and Reni hat. From our closeness in childhood, I'd drifted away from my cousins a little during the 80s, me with my Chelsea boots and Creation singles, them with their stonewashed denim and Ford Capris. But now, up and down the country as the 90s begin, Arab embraces Jew, Ulsterman hugs Fenian and the lambs bleat happily as they arch their backs into the lions. Former cardigan-wearing indie kids find themselves in dancefloor scrums with the side partings and slip-ons who once pummelled them in the hallways of the school. *Come together.*

One night at the Sub Club, lost in Finitribe's '101', Gary and I see each other through the clouds of steam and sweat across the packed dancefloor: both of us full of drink, sulphate and ecstasy. We point, laughing, as we stumble towards each other and embrace in the smoke-machine haze, strobing lights, sound – *'bass can you hear me?*

Loud and clear' – deafening from the bins. Gary grabs the back of my neck, puts his mouth to my ear, and pulls me into him as he shouts, *'Ma brother in arms, ma brother in arms . . .'*

I can still feel his skin against mine. The smell of his aftershave. The bristle of his cheek. How fiercely we hugged, both of us utterly gone in the new togetherness.

It becomes clear to me that Shades is a star in this new world. Handsome, with a succession of beautiful rave girlfriends, a great dancer, funny. For a moment, his reckless bravery, his foolhardiness, his willingness to do anything to stand out, these have all been subsumed in impressions and jokes and a keep-the-party-burning spirit that sees him the life and soul into the early hours of the morning, into the dawn of the next day. And then the next. He is a player now, and I am his chubbier, uncool elder brother. For the first time I hear myself being defined by my relationship to him, being referred to as 'Shades' big brother'. One night I sit down in the corner booth of the Sub Club, taking a seat just vacated by Shades, and Vouchers, who had just been talking to him, turns around to resume their conversation. He reels back in horror. 'Fuck!' he says, looking at me. 'It's like Shades was still there but he'd been blown up with a bicycle pump!' Everything is suddenly awash with Es and acid and speed and cannabis. Cannabis! Once the preserve of guys like Craig Russell's older brother – the guys with the ZOFO posters and the patchouli oil reek drifting from their bedrooms – suddenly *everyone* is 'smoking draw' all the time. You almost expect to pop home for a visit and find dad in dungarees, tossing over the Rizlas with a 'skin up, wee boy', as he cues up *Herb Albert's Utah Saints*.

In the early hours of one Sunday morning, at an after-party in someone's flat in Glasgow, me and Keith Martin are stretched out on the carpet, spangled, our pupils the size of chocolate buttons, watching everyone dancing and hugging. 'Do you think it's better now?' I ask him, groping to try and understand something.

'Eh?'

'The way things are. You know, a few years back it was all fringes and The Smiths and sitting around in our bedrooms. Is this better?'

'Fuck, Ah don't know, John,' Keith says, seriously, taking a proffered joint and dragging deeply as he looks at the roaring, dancing scrum. He turns his green-eyed gaze on me, thoughtful, serious as he gestures to the room. 'I mean, every cunt's up the pole now.'

It might feel excessive, or hackneyed, to say it today, but as the 90s begin it feels much like it must have done when The Beatles arrived in the summer of 1963: the famous black and white into Technicolor shift. People change their clothes, their hair, their careers. Our cousin Kevin quits his job and opens a record shop in Glasgow, Bomba, on West George Street, just a few hundred yards away from Splash One Happening, where we'd spent those Sunday nights in striped tops and cardigans, frugging to The 13th Floor Elevators. Now Kevin's selling the same kids the tunes they're hearing on Friday and Saturday nights, pumped up the pole on pills. People are setting up record labels or running nightclubs. Bricklayers become DJs and hairdressers become promoters. In Britain in the early 90s the nightclub flyer industry probably has a GDP close to that of Wales. But some people can't manage DJs or design flyers or run events or write fanzines. They have to find other ways to take their place at the table . . .

For Shades, like so many others, the weekend has grown to encompass Thursday through Monday. Weed smoking has become a daily thing. And a regular job gradually becomes something of an

174

encumbrance, as old-fashioned as barrel making or loom weaving. One night, in the pub down in Irvine, someone on our table is talking about these new pills he had at the weekend. 'Kinda like Doves, ken? Really strong, kicked right in fast, man. Aye, Ah goat them aff that boy whit's-his-name. He's a runner for wee Shades.'

'Sorry, what did you say?'

'They're like Doves?'

'No, about Shades?'

'Aye, he's a runner for Shades.'

Hang on – my wee brother has *a runner*?

If you have a runner, I wonder, how far up the food chain does that put you? *The stone goes through the window, the shoes go into the pond, the breadknife is at the wrists and Gary is a bad wee stick.*

Gary is fired from his job at Fullarton Fabrications, for driving a forklift truck without a licence or permission. He claims that 'the foreman telt me tae dae it!' But there's the possibility that Shades had simply been showing off, doing something none of the other boys had the balls to do. Up in the attic bedroom at mum and dad's house, his posters for club nights at the Metro and the Pleasure Dome hang where my punk ones once had. He isn't really working, but he seems to be OK for money. Mainly his new lifestyle is consuming his energy. There's very little sleep between Friday and Monday – often he won't come home – and then there are the midweek comedowns, the sullen depressions, the silences and irrational rages. All of this has coincided almost perfectly with dad's retirement. So they're both in the house a lot, and while there's the odd respite – still the garbage Saturday night TV, or the two of them hunkered over tinned spaghetti on toast in front of *Neighbours* in the afternoon – tensions begin to worsen. Dad has little understanding of, or sympathy with, the world of banging tunes and DJ sets and the whole 'whatever you do just make sure whatever you're doing makes you happy' philosophy of the times. He cannot comprehend why, when he should be out looking for a job and finding a job, Gary is regularly coming home at dawn and clanking up the metal ladder to the attic, where he'll sleep the entire day away, cocooning himself until early evening, when he emerges, all dressed up again, to grab a long-necked Budweiser from the fridge, twist the cap off it, and get on the phone to make plans for the night, a night that, like the last one, will end with his Wallabees on the stepladder somewhere around dawn. All too regularly, it begins to go a little something like this . . .

Gary, coming in the front door in the late morning, swaying, reeking of drink, his eyes glazed, still high. Dad, coming out of the living room – 'Where the hell have you been out to till this time?'

'Ach, gies peace.' Gary starts to head up the stairs, dad following.

'On a Monday morning, Gary! Ye should be out looking fur a bloody job!' Gary's feet trudging upstairs, heading for the dark and cool and quiet of the attic. 'Look at the state o' ye, boy!'

'Aye aye.'

'Ah mean it. Ye can get oot o' this hoose if ye think all yer gaunnae do is go oot drinking aw night and sleeping aw day.'

'Ah fucking will then!'

'HEY! You watch your language, boy!'

'LEE ME ALANE!'

Dad is up the stairs now, getting in his face. 'Yer jist a bloody bum, Gary!'

176

'GET TAE FUCK!'

'GET OOT O' THIS HOOSE!'

Dad grabs him. Gary pushes back. They tussle. Gary breaks free. And then his feet, clanging on the aluminium stepladder, the ladder dad screwed into place nearly twenty years before, all full of hope for the future, for his young family, for his sons. For the son who is now a dangerous stranger to him, whose feet stomp around overhead. Dad shouts up at the Artex ceiling – 'Yer a waste o' space so ye are! Ye'll end up in the bloody Bar-L!'

'FUCK OFF!'

The trapdoor cracks down. Dad stands there, steadying himself on the little ledge at the top of the stairs, panting, shaking, saying to himself, 'That bloody boy.' In the blackness of the windowless attic, Gary gets undressed, swallows Temazepam, and climbs into bed. Downstairs, mum cries.

'Plastics, Ben'

Thirty miles away, in Glasgow, driven by the zest of now being a 'mature student', I put in long hours in the library and finally graduate with a First in the summer of 1991. Mum cries. Dad says, 'Ah'm awfy proud o' ye, son.' There isn't much from Gary. Because the summer has brought a rift between us, after Stephanie and I got engaged and, in a break from tradition, I failed to ask my brother to be my best man. Shades cuts me off and does not come to the wedding. So I sigh and tut and shake my head as I hear of his latest outrages and transgressions from Linda, safe with my fiancée and our mortgage, far away in the big city. But, in truth, like Shades, I'm kind of rudderless myself. For graduation has brought a paralysis: Benjamin Braddock, at the bottom of the pool, in his mask. I'm not sure I want to go down the obvious route that is open to you when you get a First in English Literature: academia. Because, before you even get to all that, there's the idea of spending another three years near penniless while you do your PhD. I'm twenty-four now and I've never really earned a penny in my life. It's been two years at university, two in the band, two at university again. What I'm really into is the idea of finally making some money . . .

Oddly, and this self is truly unrecognisable to me now, my degree secures me milk-round interviews with a few merchant banks: Salomon Brothers, Lehman Brothers, Credit Suisse. It soon becomes clear that their trainee jobs call for: a) a head for figures, b) 7am starts and c) fourteen-hour days. It really does seem like work. I am lazy and yet avaricious – characteristics that will make me an ideal candidate for the career that is about to unfold when, a few months after graduation, towards the end of 1991, my cousin Kevin and I go for a drink at Bar Ten on Mitchell Lane, near his record shop, Bomba, on West George Street. He has a proposition. Business is brisk at the shop and he's opened two more branches in Ayr and Inverness. He now wants to start a label, putting out the kind of records he's selling. At this brief juncture in history – before there will soon be more people making records than there are buying them – a happening dance label can shift anywhere between 5,000 and 20,000 copies of a release, figures that would put you comfortably in the Top 10 today. Kevin knows I was kind of around the music business, with the band, and he asks if I know much about things like distribution and getting press coverage and stuff. These are terms I'd heard Jeff Barrett use. I'd heard the terms, but I didn't really know what they meant. Kevin is picking my brains, but there really isn't that much to pick. 'Yeah, sure,' I lie. 'I know how all that stuff works.'

I start working for Kevin in a kind of press officer/label manager/ general dogsbody capacity. The money is minimal, but it's immediately more fun than Credit Suisse looked like being. Anyway, I reason, it'll lead to something bigger.

'He didnae want to worry all of you . . .'

There was never any family summit. The five of us never sat down around a table while mum and dad laid out the options, the scenarios. We were just told, matter-of-factly, early in 1993, that dad had cancer 'in the gut'. But they'd caught it early enough, he was going to get chemo and it would all work out. We weren't to worry. 'I feel fine,' dad said. The tension between Shades and dad doesn't completely disappear, but it does get turned down a notch. Another upside of dad's illness is a healing of the eighteen-month silence Gary has extended towards me. 'It's too long for bad blood between brothers, Gary,' dad tells him. 'Ye need tae make it up with John.' And we do, we get past it, and both of us return to throwing ourselves into our respective roles in the UK dance scene – me trying to get records written about in the music press, and Gary doing his part to make sure the intended audience for these records hears them in what might be called a 'receptive' state of mind. Meanwhile, in the background, dad quietly gets thinner and yellower. Were mum and dad confident he would 'beat' the cancer, as the tabloids say? Or were they just quietly joining the right queue? Many years later, I ask mum if they deliberately sugarcoated the situation for us, especially for Linda, who was only eighteen at the time. 'Maybe a wee bit, son. He didnae want to worry all of you.'

And so life went on.

Writing #3

I make another attempt at a novel around now. Horror is the chosen genre this time, as I sit in front of the second-hand Amstrad computer that has replaced the Olivetti. The emerald-green screen, the type glowing through as though coming from beneath the glass of a whisky bottle. As far as I can recall the book was a kind of James Herbert/Stephen King mash-up about giant mutant amphibians breeding under the floor-boards of a mental hospital (?!) But Mr Niven was still confused about the perspective from which to tell his story and once again the thing spluttered out after a hundred or so pages. But, again, I was very much in thrall to the experience of doing it. Part of me knew I was only playing at being a writer; still, I loved being alone at the desk, watching the paragraphs grow, the satisfying way the pages spooled from the printer at the end of the day. I loved it in the same way I loved being in the university library late at night, surrounded by books and folders, notepads and pens. (Even today, when I see this scene generically represented in a Hollywood film – the hero or heroine alone in the vast public library, with their yellow legal pad under the glow of the inevitable green banker's lamp – a yearning part of me cries out with Liz Lemon's *I want to go to there*.) I didn't yet know that playing at something was an essential step on the road to becoming it. I didn't know either that loving doing it meant that I already had an essential component of the writer's make-up in my toolbox: you are most fully alive when alone.

It was in one of the small rooms on the upstairs gallery of the circular reading room, studying for my finals in the spring of 1991, that I accidentally came across a paperback copy of *Adventures in the Screen Trade* by William Goldman, the legendary screenwriter's account of the years in Hollywood when he wrote *Butch Cassidy and the Sundance Kid*, *Marathon Man* and *All the President's Men*. I was spellbound by it, although it would be years before I truly understood what Goldman meant by his maxim 'screenplays are structure'. One of Goldman's other catechisms was the famed 'no one knows anything', used to describe the non-processes of Hollywood, the way people will confidently proclaim the western dead as a commercial genre and then must recalibrate their position as *Unforgiven* cruises to glory, or the way the can't-miss blockbuster with A-list stars barely opens while the indie picture with a cast of unknowns breaks box-office records.

Soon, I will begin to get an abject lesson in 'no one knows anything'.

'Drive safe'

I go down to Irvine to see dad, just before Easter. I'm off to London with Kevin again. Then Steph and I will be travelling to the other end of the country, to Teignmouth in Devon, to spend the holiday with her parents. Dad is sitting up in bed. He's been increasingly unwell, tired, taking to bed more and more. His hair is still unaffected by the chemo, the same thick grey it's been since he was in his late fifties, but there's a yellowish tint to his skin now and his temples are hollowing from weight loss. But still, he insists he's 'fine'. The brown tubs of pills next to the water glass, the portable TV showing snooker,

181

the ever-present blue-on-white pack of Embassy Regal with the disposable plastic lighter on top of it. The purple glass, dimpled ashtray.

'How do you feel, dad?'

'Ach, jist tired, John.'

He asks me to unplug something from the plugboard by the bed and plug something else in for him. I accidentally unplug the bedside radio/alarm clock, meaning that the time will have to be reset. He snaps at me, and we have a stupid, petty squabble.

'OK, fine. I'll see you after the holidays, dad,' I sigh. Still, I kiss his forehead on my way out, as I always do.

'Aye, cheerio, son. Drive safe.'

I leave him in bed, watching snooker on the TV in the faded blue paisley pyjamas he'd owned since the early 70s. The clack of balls from the tiny speaker. The cigarette smouldering between his fingers like a fuse.

Aw That Shakespeare Way

'Have at thou, Garfunkel!'

Shades shouts it again. He's standing on the table of the pub off Shepherd's Bush Green, miming thrusting an invisible sword at a shadow enemy, as everyone falls around, broken with laughter. There is me and Keith and Andy O'Hagan and Larry and Tony and Peter Trodden and Tud (my wife Charlotte, many years later: 'Why do you call your friend that awful name?' 'It's short for Tudhope. Alan Tudhope. It's his name.' A pause. 'Oh, I thought you were all calling him *Turd*.') and a good few others. Soul to Soul's 'Back To Life' shakes the room.

In truth, making everyone collapse with laughter is not a hugely difficult task at this point: we have all been up all night, at various raves and parties, and have coalesced here to begin the second day of drinking, or, rather, to continue the first. From the pub to the club to the after-party, to the after-after-party, then back to the pub in the afternoon. In five years the price of those white pills has collapsed – from twenty pounds to fifteen to a tenner. It's no longer a single pill savoured all night, *bags* of them make the rounds now. And then there's something else that's crept in: the sustaining hourly, then half-hourly, trips to the toilet with the wraps of cocaine. The invincibility of your twenties, the marathons of narcotics and drink that would be hospitalising – *hospice-ising* – today.

'*Have at thou, Garfunkel!*'

The staff are shouting at Shades to get down now, to behave.

Kevin and I are in London doing Bomba stuff, meeting Amato who distribute our records, the three singles we've released over the course of late 1992/1993. Shades and his mates are down on one of their regular trips to experience some of that London clubbing. His table-top performance has been inspired by overhearing a shameful conversation between me and O'Hagan. My degree is only a couple of years behind me, and Andy has just started as an assistant editor at the *London Review of Books*. So somehow we've got onto *literature* of all things, sleepless and bent on chemicals. Shades catches a snippet of whatever we're gibbering about and lasers in – 'Whit kind o' holy fucking pish are you pair o' benders talking aboot? Fucking aw that Shakespeare way fur fuck sake?' He slams his pint down and gains the tabletop.

'*Aww – have at thou, Garfunkel!*'

He slashes at the air with his mind-rapier. Whether Gary was thinking of Paul Simon's former singing partner or the London restaurant chain is lost to history. But the fact that he has boiled all of Shakespeare down to this particular name ends all of us that afternoon. We watch him caper like a madman, his face beaming, delighted with himself as he shouts, '*Have at thou, Garfunkel!*' over and over again.

I see my brother still: silhouetted against the spring sunshine flooding through the windows, his Timberlands kicking a jig among the rattling empties as the barman shouts another weary warning. I

184

see Keith laughing, reaching the certain point of mania Keith would sometimes reach when he *really* laughed, a kind of wide-eyed, this-can't-be-happening disbelief, his grin huge, every gleaming tooth visible, his shoulders shaking, but the sound yet to emerge, still pregnant within him. That was how we were all laughing with Shades that afternoon, everyone sleepless and mad and drunk and pilled-up, primed, begging for this kind of hysteria. And what a bequest, Gary, Keith.

These are the things the friends and family who die too soon really leave us, if we are very lucky: an inheritance of comedy with an incredibly powerful half-life. One that, thirty or forty years later, will cause the grin to spread over your face when you're stuck in traffic, when you're putting the bananas on the conveyor belt and reaching for the divider to separate your purchases from the scattered tins in front. When you're sitting at your desk, typing, tiny specks of snow drifting by your window, like pieces of your past, falling silently from the sky.

'Tea or coffee?'

Three days later, Friday, 30 April 1993, Steph and I are in Devon, in Teignmouth, where she grew up, where her parents still live, in a large, high house overlooking the English Channel.

Early that morning, first thing, we go down into the town, where I get a haircut as soon as the barber opens. We wander the streets for a bit – the café, the bookshop – before heading back to her parents' place around 11am. Tony and Margaret are nice people, decent and kind. Being middle-class (self-made, from Sheffield. Tony worked his way up from bank clerk to bank manager, to bank inspector) they run cooler than my Ayrshire kin, coming across as a little stiff and reserved in comparison. They have endearing English habits, like asking 'do you want a drink?' when they actually mean a hot beverage, a usage that stopped me in my tracks the first time I heard it, at maybe ten o'clock in the morning. *Woah,* I briefly thought, before realising they meant tea, *these guys run hard.* Tony listens to classical music and has a baby grand piano in the living room. They go rambling. Their family gatherings do not descend into whisky-soaked routs. There is no Uncle Drew pointing at an empty space on the wall at three in the morning and screaming, 'DO YOU SEE ANY SUFFERING CLOCKS IN THIS HOOSE?' They are unlikely to shout, 'YE DAFT HOORMASTER!' at a professional golfer missing a putt on television. We walk into the kitchen to find Margaret and Tony both standing there, both rigid, looking at me intently, even fearfully, as I come through the door. Margaret is wringing her hands, almost trembling.

My first thought is that I have gone much, much too far at the barber's (Alan Patterson, stuffing that fist into his mouth, the old boy's baleful *'Jesus Christ, son'*) and my hand flies to my hair, patting the sides. 'Is it too sh–'

But it's not the hair.

'John,' Tony says. 'Your mum called. It . . . it's your dad.'

Your mind spirals upwards through the degrees. He's taken a turn for the worse. He's in hospital. He's in intensive care. He's . . .

'I'm so sorry – he's dead,' Tony says.

Your sticky wee hands help me get a good grip . . . a PUNK ROCK CONCERT IN MA BLOODY GARAGE? . . . turn yer shoulders now,

keep your head down . . . AM AH NO DEAD WITH IT! Night, night,
son . . . cheerio, son . . . drive safe.

'Would you like a drink?' Margaret says.

I nod, my legs going.

'Tea or coffee?'

I just look at Stephanie. She fetches the whisky.

Mum answers, 'Ahh, ahh, John, son.' She must suck air in before she can speak, like a child crying. The words gradually come through the tears and she tells me what happened . . .

He'd been getting increasingly weak over the last forty-eight hours. She'd rung the doctor yesterday afternoon, saying he couldn't seem to get enough oxygen, couldn't catch his breath. She thought he might need a blood transfusion or something. The doctor didn't think it would help. Then, last night, as it got dark outside, his breathing started to get shallower and shallower. Around midnight, he started slipping in and out of consciousness. Although breathless, he doesn't seem scared. (*The shift into the present tense here, dad. Trying to keep you around just a wee bit longer.*) But he knows what is happening to him because he tells her that he loves her very much and that she should marry again.

'*You're still young,*' dad says, '*don't waste your life.*' The older I get, the more this feels like the very definition of love: the wish that it should continue without you. And, finally, the very last thing he will ever say to her, thirty years after they met – '*Look after the three of them.*'

Just before 1am, dad dies.

Mum screams for Gary, sleeping above them, and, moments later, his feet come rattling down the metal ladder from the attic. He shoulders

187

his way bleary-eyed into the bedroom to see mum cradling him, sobbing as she says, *'Aww, John. Aww, John. Don't go! Don't leave me!'*

The doctor puts the time of death at 1am on 30 April and will list the primary cause as 'carcinoma of the oesophagus' with a secondary of 'myocardial ischemia'. The cancer, causing heart failure. (Why had mum waited until morning to call me? 'You were five hundred miles away, son. By the time the doctor had finished it was the middle of the night. What good would it have done?') The only Niven child there when our father dies, Gary climbs onto the bed and buries his face in his dad's neck as he starts to cry too. I often picture him at that moment: shaking and weeping as the chain reaction that will power him into the next phase of his life starts up.

Lee us alane! Lee us alane!

No – don't leave us, please don't leave us . . . fuck off . . . I hate you. I don't . . . I didn't mean it . . . just wake up, just for a minute . . . I want to . . . I'm sorry . . . I'm sorry . . . I . . .

The unsaid.

I come into the living room: Aunt Bell and Aunt Emily. Uncle Alec and Uncle Drew. Linda, just nineteen, looks at me, wide-eyed. She had been up very late, at a party at her friend's house, and had crawled into bed just before dawn when, a couple of hours later, Uncle Drew had arrived at the door unannounced to collect her, to tell her that, just around the corner, her father lay dead. Mum sees me enter the crowded room and tries to stand up from the sofa. In a reverse of that moment with Shades and me in the Sub Club, it looks as though someone has found a valve somewhere and let half the air out of her. She seems *tiny*, desiccated, still in deep shock, with a thousand-yard stare, like she doesn't quite know where she is. But she manages to focus, catching her breath as I come towards her. (Perhaps, I reflect later, my likeness to my dad almost too much to be borne at that moment.) We both say the same thing through our tears – 'Happy Birthday.'

I find Shades in the kitchen, a lager in one hand, a lit Kensitas Club in the other. He's staring, vacant and hollow, red-eyed, and it takes him a moment to recognise me. 'Awright, wee boy?' he says as we hug. Then – 'Do ye want to come and see him?' Shades leads the way upstairs, to where the tiny walk-through room has been hard pressed into one final, even more unlikely, incarnation: a funeral parlour.

Dad lies in the open coffin, feet towards the door, so that on entering I get a view directly up the twin barrels of his vast nostrils. He has been dead for less than thirty-six hours and the death chemistry has not fully transfigured him yet. He looks like at any moment he might sit up and bark for the TV remote, or shout at you for unplugging the wrong thing. It is the fourth time I have seen a dead body – both of his parents, mum's father – but I have never touched one before. I reach out and press the back of my hand to his cheek. As expected, it is cold, waxy, but I can still feel the sandpaper rasp of his stubble, the hairs that felt as thick as the bristles on a paintbrush when we were kids. He's wearing one of his golf sweaters, a Pringle, and an open-necked shirt. The smells of who he was – Old Spice and tobacco and Swarfega and Famous Grouse – are still there. I kiss his forehead, cold as the window of a jet, his hair still smelling exactly as it has all my life, and I rest my head on his chest and break down.

★ ★ ★

Late that night, I am lying in bed in my old room, Linda sleeping next door with mum, when I hear Gary's voice coming softly through the thin partition wall. He is talking to the man who put up the wall, back in 1973, the man in the coffin. I cannot make out the words, but the tone is clear. It is contrition. It is all getting said now, finally, through tears and catching breaths. But it is getting said to a corpse.

And the price for the delay will be steep. Ruinous.

At the end of the year, at Christmas, Stephanie will give Gary the framed picture of dad in the RAF, in North Africa. The howl of anguish. Then the wailing run from the living room, down the short hallway and through the tiny kitchen. (We know this run well, mum. *Who loves ya, baby?*) And then his fists, driving over and over into the wooden wall of the garage, the knuckles splitting open, the wood splintering, the unsaid becoming the only thing getting said, over and over and over, for the rest of his life.

I speak at dad's funeral. I still have the notes for that speech nearly thirty years later, scribbled on the back of a manila envelope in pale, faded blue ballpoint. I talked about golf and love and the thirty years he and mum had together, and, at one point, I said something glib about how I can't be too sad because – in all the random chaos of the cosmos – I was very lucky to have known him at all. The fatuous idiot that I was at twenty-seven. Christ, what did I know? I look back at us now, at the little family on the front pew, in the functional crematorium. Linda, still a teenager, bewildered, mum in shock, and Shades, fidgeting in the oversized suit, bought the day before, pain and rage and regret behind the blue eyes, the eyes that dart and flicker constantly, self-conscious and guilty. Later, we scatter his ashes along the first hole at Ravenspark, beginning on the tee box, the one we

190

had stepped onto so many times with him, every time with the turf springy beneath your spikes, offering the promise of a fresh start, of perfection. Gary, Linda and I run down the fairway throwing great handfuls of him into the air, getting him on our clothes, in our faces, in our hair, our lungs. Full of him.

The following year, 1994, I will go back to London.

Gary will go to hell.

PART FOUR

Thursday, 2 September 2010

I wake up early, just after dawn, back in my teenage bedroom at the age of forty-four. Well, I'm in half of it. The partition wall was knocked down a few years back, mum returning the house to its original two-bedroom configuration. The strange, universal sense of depersonalisation this brings, the peeling away of adulthood, of all you have accumulated since you left a room like this room. All the plans you made in here, in the crucible of your adolescence. All the anxieties and insecurities you tried to work your way through. You can feel them all gathering, the person you were back then, trying to seep back into your bones. The curtains are thin and, at night, the streetlight seeps in, the same streetlight that lit the thousands of nights I spent in here, hunched over the record player, the *NME*, the guitar, dreaming of being somewhere else, someone else. The bed, the room, the house, the town – they all feel much, much too small now. I lie in bed thinking about the little warren of rooms around me as I yawn and stretch, Linda still asleep in mum's bed next door, mum, up for a while now, shuffling around downstairs, making more coffee, turning up Radio 2. I am already wanting all of this to end, to move on to the next phase: grief, mourning, whatever.

I want to get in the hire car and drive to Glasgow Airport. I want the attendant to bring my Bloody Mary as we fly back to Heathrow, away from all this mess, away from all the stuff that you can't leave behind. But we must go back to the hospital.

So we go.

We meet the latest in a long line of doctors, this one a senior consultant, who tells us that they have finally performed an MRI scan and that the results are 'not very encouraging' but that they're going to 'wait just a little bit longer'.

'Can we see the scan, please?' I ask.

He hesitates. 'I don't know if that would help you.'

'Why not?'

'Well, would you even know what you're looking at, Mr Niven?'

'Of course not. You can explain it to me.'

'I don't think I can,' he says.

'Why not?'

'Umm, patient confidentiality,' he says, incredibly.

He's reaching. There is almost a question mark left hanging in the air after that 'confidentiality'.

And a voice in my head says, *'That's enough of this nonsense.'*

I take him, lightly, by the elbow and walk him a few paces away from my mother and sister. 'The patient,' I say, nodding towards Gary in the bed, my voice very quiet and calm (my voice icy, a bad sign – in his diaries Alan Clark describes this as being 'just one step away from bellowing with rage') 'is unconscious and, as you just implied, unlikely to ever regain consciousness.' I am speaking through my gritted bottom teeth now, just like dad when in fury. '*If* he does, he's going to be severely brain-damaged.

196

I want to know exactly what's happened to my brother so we can explain it to my mum. I want someone to show me the scan and walk me through exactly what he's done to himself. Do you understand?'

By the end of this little speech, I am doing talking-to-a-child cadence. We face off. He's angry, this guy. Unused to being spoken to like this. After a moment he says, 'I don't know if I can make that decision.'

'Then go and get the person who can.'

Another beat. He holds my gaze. 'Just a minute,' he says.

He leaves. It's real, then. The growing feeling I've had since I got here – of closing ranks and protecting flanks. Of people running scared.

A few minutes pass with the now utterly familiar sound: the steady hiss and click of the ventilator as it makes his chest rise and fall, those pale blue coils on the monitor screens, the smell of disinfectant. The three-day stubble on Gary's face. His eyes still gummed shut. The red marks at the corners of his mouth, from the tubes, from where mum keeps wiping away the saliva that crusts there. Mum is holding his hand again as she talks to him. Telling him about our night, about what we had for dinner, about when we got up that morning, about what went on with *PopMaster*.

The consultant finally returns. 'Mr Niven?'

'What the hell goes on in your bloody heid, Gary?'

I remembered dad asking this, more than once, after whatever fresh outrage had been committed. Here it was, dad. All laid out like a split cauliflower. We're in a small cubicle off the ICU. Up on the lightbox on the wall are the scans of Gary's brain, bone-white standing out against smoked grey. The consultant's silver pen glides across the scans as he explains the clinical picture. Fintan's instinct had been correct:

197

Gary has effectively caused a monumental stroke. All the upper brain functions – memory, perception, motor skills, cognition – have been wiped out. Logic and reason are gone. (Again, and God help me, Linda, but how would we tell?) So, there's no other way to ask it. 'Why are we keeping him alive?'

'Because we cannot say with total certainty that Gary is technically brain-dead.'

Again, Fintan had anticipated and explained this. There might be a chance of him being able to breathe on his own if some of the brain stem's core functions were still intact. Based on his complete non-responses to stimuli so far, this is unlikely, but the only way to properly find out would mean taking him off the ventilator and seeing what happens. They will need our permission to do this and the doctor still wants to wait another twenty-four hours.

'What might change?' I ask.

He looks at me and says, 'You're a very inquisitive person.' This is not meant as a compliment.

I take a deep breath and say, 'As you might be, if your brother had walked into a hospital perfectly healthy and found himself a vegetable the next day.'

'Yes,' he says, snapping the lightbox off, his own temper showing. 'But another way to look at it would be that if this had happened to him somewhere else and he wasn't already in a hospital, then he'd definitely be dead.'

This certainly strikes me as what, a couple of years from now, will become known as 'a hot take'. I don't know what I can even begin to say in response to that, so I settle for my own curt 'thank you for your time' and go off to find Linda.

198

I take her outside, where I smoke, and we discuss how to break all this to mum. Linda has a fifteen-month-old daughter at home. She needs to get back to Glasgow. We agree that, after I tell mum what the MRI shows, I should, as gently as possible, try to steer her towards the idea of agreeing to turn the ventilator off and seeing if Gary can breathe on his own. We go back and collect her – she leaves Gary with a kiss on the forehead and the promise that she will see him later – and I drop Linda at the train station then drive us on down to the beach park.

We go for a walk along the harbour. The fine weather continues, and today might well be the most perfect so far. It's around twenty-two degrees, the sunshine sparkling across the still water at the mouth of the river Irvine. The ancient, rusted blue crane is still here, the one that we used to dive off when we were boys, as dad had before us. Across the river the sand dunes and sea grass stretch off past Bogside and on to Ardeer, to the munitions factory where dad's fiancée died in that explosion nearly seventy years ago. And if that explosion hadn't happened, then I wouldn't be here and neither would Gary and so on and so on. I look at mum looking at the sea, and I wonder what she's remembering.

Back in the mid- to late 70s, during the long summer holidays, she would bring the three of us and our King Charles Spaniel Candy down here nearly every day, a two-and-a-half-mile walk with a toddler, two small boys, a dog and the beach bag over her shoulder, crammed with towels and buckets and spades. Her tartan flask of coffee. The Tupperware box with ham and tomato sandwiches, the bread damp from the tomatoes, flecked with sand by the time we ate them. The walk would take us from our house, along Elmbank Terrace, past the church and then by the shops on Caldon Road. Back then the newsagent on Caldon Road sold toys and groceries, ham freshly sliced in the big, terrifying machine, sweets from huge glass jars. There was translucent yellow flypaper across the bottom half of the windows and in summer scores of the dead insects lay at the bottom. One hot day, not long after we had moved to Livingstone Terrace – making me seven or eight, Gary five or six – we had stood gazing longingly through that window at the Airfix models of World War Two aircraft while mum was inside shopping. As we gazed the shopkeeper's hands came into view and lifted two 1/72 scale models – a Spitfire and a Messerschmitt – out of the display. Some kid had just scored big, I remember thinking. When mum came out of the shop, she handed us the models. We hadn't even asked for them. We didn't have a lot of money and these were expensive gifts for us, the kind of thing usually reserved for birthdays or Christmas. I asked her why she had bought them for us.

'Because you were being good boys and hadn't asked for anything.'

I see Gary still, hugging mum in gratitude, his arms wrapped around her legs in the sunshine on Caldon Road, his head nestling into her hip. It is one of those random memories of parental love and kindness that causes your heart to flex in your chest all these years later, a moment that you know will very likely be somewhere amongst your last thoughts. Is it somewhere amongst his now? Are there any thoughts left? Or are they all leaving him, swirling like a galaxy of stars circling a black hole and then vanishing, the memories of a lifetime crackling like the screen of an old television set, pinprick pixels disappearing into a white spot in the centre, then slowly fading away to nothing? Have they already left? Is his mind already a dead screen, the screen of the portable television

200

after it toppled backwards to the bedroom floor, the tubes smashed, the circuit boards burned out, the glass cold to the touch, not even the Velcro crackle of the residue of electricity as you draw your hand across it. From the newsagent we'd continue along Quarry Road, past the playing fields, past the Wan Lung and the Gay Bogs, then across the high street and down East Road, past the pitch-and-putt course and across the river on the green metal bridge at the Low Green, past the sawmill where our Uncle Sid worked, past Fullarton Parish Church, where our parents had been married, and finally onto Montgomery Street, the final stretch towards the beach. The newsagent, the Gay Bogs, the pitch-and-putt and the sawmill and dad are all long gone now as I sit with mum in the warm sun on a bench overlooking the mouth of the river, with the ghosts of childhood all around: Gary and me running whooping into that water, Linda singing to herself as she filled and emptied her wee plastic bucket with sand, as she patted at it with her plastic spade, Candy whimpering in the shade of the windbreak, her golf-ball eyes pleading in the heat, mum slathered in Ambre Solaire, frowning into her fat Mills & Boon. She was in her early thirties back then. Her husband had a good job and a car. Her children were all healthy. It was, I now understand, the happiest time of her life. The woman next to me is sixty-seven. Her husband is dead. Her youngest son is neither dead nor alive, floating in purgatory eight miles east of us.

'Mum, listen,' I say, taking her hand.

The night before, Linda and I sat up after mum went to bed, making our way through a bottle of red and talking Shades.

'New Year was always a bad time for him,' Linda said. 'The one before dad died, 1992, mum and dad were away, I'm still living at home, and I decided I was going to have a New Year's Eve party. Gary was in a flat at the time, nearby, around Martin Avenue? Anyway, he hears about the party, comes around to the house and says, "Naw, you're no doing that. The place could get wrecked." I tried to explain that it wouldn't be a big do, all our mutuals would be there – Peter Trodden, Tony Scott, David and Kevin, that kind of thing – but no sale. Gary is adamant I'm not having a party, and I'm nineteen at this point, so I'm like, "You're not the boss of me." So the argument escalates, he's in my face, screaming at me, shoving me, pushing his finger in my chest, and then he storms out the front door, he's walking across the street, heading back to his flat, and I shout after him, "Wanker!" And I remember really clearly, he stops, turns around, and walks very slowly and deliberately back towards the house – I've no idea why I didn't just lock the front door – and he comes in, shoves me down in the kitchen and just starts battering my face off the floor. Then he leaves. I'm crying, a mess. But I phone a few of my pals and they're like "fuck him", so we go ahead and have the party. Shades rings the house while it's going on and Tony Scott answers and calms him down, tells him everything's fine. Later, Shades arrives. He rocks up with these three girls – rough, hard-looking girls that no one knew – and all of them are jellied out of their minds, just wrecked. One of them ends up sitting on that wee nest of side tables mum had and just smashing them to bits.'

She sighed. Sipped her wine.

'You know, after all his shite about the house getting wrecked, the only trouble caused was by him and these lunatics he'd started to run around with.'

We sat with our glasses in the tangerine flicker of the living-flame gas fire, that has replaced the coal-effect electric fire, that replaced the coal fire. These four walls we grew up within.

'The next year, 1993, the first new year after dad died, mum went away to a hotel with Aunt Emily, and Shades is back living at home and he decides *he's* going to have a party. I came around quite late on, and it's scary. I mean there's the Davidsons there, Jock, all that lot. I come into the hall and see that the living-room door's been smashed to pieces, like someone's taken an axe to it. I come down the hall, trying to find Shades, and the kitchen window has a black binbag taped over it. It's been smashed too. Finally, I see Shades, in the corner of the kitchen. His face is all cut to bits, bleeding. A big gash across his nose. Turns out he'd gone berserk and just smashed his head through the window. All his mates think it's hilarious. All jellied off their nuts. Me and my pals just wound up leaving. It was starting to get dark, the people he was running with.'

'It all got exponentially worse after dad died, didn't it?'

'He'd start talking some nights about how he was going to go over the golf course with a sleeping bag, to spend the night with dad, on the first hole, you know? I don't think he ever did it.'

'What was the other time? With the gun?'

'That was the following New Year, 1994. Mum's away again, and Jim is staying over, so the two of us are sleeping in mum and dad's bed. Well, obviously it's just mum's bed at that point. I get woken up at four in the morning by Shades. He bursts in the bedroom and tells us, "Get the fuck out, I'm sleeping here."

'"But, Gary," I said, "there's two of us. This is the only double bed. You've got your own bedroom upstairs."

'"Get out ma dad's bed," he says. "I'm sleeping there." I remember he definitely said that – *my dad's bed*. He said, "I'll give you ten minutes," and stormed off. We fell back asleep. The next thing I know, he's back in the room screaming, "GET THE FUCK OUT! NOW!" I jump up and he's standing there pointing a bloody gun at us.'

'Jesus.'

'I swear to God. I mean, I don't know if it's an air pistol or a real gun or whatever, but I start screaming, "OK! OK, Gary!" He leaves again, and we're getting dressed, and I decide to go downstairs and try to talk to him again. I get to the bottom of the stairs and he's coming out the living-room door.' Linda points to the door, just a few feet to my right. 'He's got a hammer in his hand. He comes towards me and brings it up over my head. I look at him, into his eyes, and they're just gone, he's on jellies, coke, whatever, and, for a second, I think – *he's going to kill me*. He looks that insane. And then I see this confusion coming across his face, like he's having a moment of thinking, *what the fuck am I doing?* And he lets the hammer drop down by his side and he starts crying and says, "Linda, I'm telling ye, jist get out of this hoose, *now*." I *run* upstairs, get Jim, and we end up walking round to his parents' in the early hours of the morning. New Year's Day, 1994.'

1994. No longer the time of ecstasy. It is the dawn of cocaine and Temazepam sweeping Scotland's club scene. The time of Black Grape's 'Tramazi Parti'.

For Shades, like many, it was all getting much darker.

There isn't a breath of wind as mum cries softly, saying the same words over and over, *'Oh, Gary, oh, son.'*

I want to say, 'It's OK, it'll be all right,' the way she had to us, countless times, in childhood. But it wasn't OK. And it wasn't going to be all right.

Looking back through my notebook from that awful week, I see that I jotted down the following, just after I told mum that the only thing keeping Gary alive was the ventilator, that he had destroyed his brain beyond all repair: '*A huge crow on a fence post near us, wings folded behind its back. Schoolmasterly. Its head clockworked around and I made eye contact. The crow as black, as mum would say, as the Earl o' Hell's waistcoat.*' I once had a colleague in the music industry who was a keen student of the numerology of nature, of things like the tidings imparted by certain birds, of certain numbers of them glimpsed together. I cannot recall any of his distinctions, but I am pretty sure that a single, staring black raven would not be among the good omens.

'No,' mum says eventually. 'He wouldn't want that. He wouldn't want to be kept alive as a vegetable.'

She says this with a certainty I find surprising, having long given up on trying to figure out Gary's take on anything. Besides, over the next few days, a lot of things that Gary wouldn't have wanted to happen are going to go right ahead and happen anyway. 'OK,' I say. 'We can talk to them about taking him off the ventilator.'

'What will that do?'

'He'll have to try and breathe on his own.'

I don't add that it's unlikely he'll be able to. And a voice that I am trying very hard not to listen to keeps saying, '*But what if he can?*'

Maximum carnage. Total chaos. The Shades Way.

All those thoughts again – the slumped figure in the wheelchair, the eyes as empty as a politician's promises. The liquidised mush being spooned in, dribbling down his chin, his bib. Twenty or thirty years of that. And, if it came to it, I wonder, pursuing the macabre fantasy as far as it will go, who would take over after mum died? It is difficult to know where the boundaries of love and duty are until you run up against them, but I know with certainty that I would not do this job. Linda, having much more in the way of the caring gene, would be a far better candidate, but I very much doubt that she would either. I picture Gary in his seventies, in the grim state nursing home, in a wheelchair parked in front of the fizzing television set, showing some game show that he cannot comprehend, the mind broken long ago, the grizzled body somehow persisting.

'Will you talk to the doctors about it, son?'

Her eyes are flickering downwards as they fill again with tears, her hands fiddling in her lap, her jaw going. For a moment, she looks like a seven-year-old who has been caught in something bad.

'I already have. They want to wait another twenty-four hours.'

It is perhaps telling that mum takes this not as a betrayal, but as positive action. We walk the rest of the way to the beach, right to the end of the short stone causeway that juts out into the sea.

The island of Arran lies straight across, the shoreline stretching away south to our left, down to Barassie, then Troon, then Ayr. To our right, to the north, lie Saltcoats, Seamill, Gourock, all these towns on the west coast of Scotland coming with their own evocations – *Arran: your stag night in 1992, Keith trying to throw your red Filas over the side of the ferry. Barassie: the Castlepark Primary School sponsored walk in '77, mum packed you a lunch, a Mermaid soft drink in a plastic pouch. Troon: pub crawl when you were sixteen, after you'd worked clearing tables in the hospitality tent at the 1982 Open, where Tom Watson won his fourth and you saw Ronnie Corbett and Telly Savalas – the breadknife. Ayr: the Subs*

206

at the Pavilion. Saltcoats: drinking in Rudi's in '83, the first time you tried
Schlitz. Seamill: the freezing saltwater pool at the Hydro hotel, where you
learned to swim with the Boy's Brigade. Gourock: Primal Scream at the Bay
Hotel in '86, Bobby's hands clasped behind his back, eyes closed, singing
'I Love You . . .'

All this flies through me in two seconds, in the time it takes to scan
the shoreline south to north. The memories that flow through you
ceaselessly, like blood, until the day you die, or until you scramble them,
wipe them like magnetic tape when you climb up on the stool in the
fluorescent cubicle, your head pounding, hot, tired and angry as you
kick it away, and then that splinter in your brain soothed forever as
the oxygen is cut off for two, three, four, six, ten minutes.

1994

Basically Happy

A fine day, the last week of May, as Shades gets off the bus at Irvine Cross and walks along the High Street towards Townhead Surgery for a GP appointment.

He's been seeing his doctor regularly over the course of the last year, as he continues to live at home with mum, as he continues to struggle with depression in the wake of dad's death. He's been prescribed Faverin, an antidepressant, but he refused to take it. Then Prozac, which he took briefly before stopping. Today his GP writes in his notes that *'his mood has deteriorated once more, and he admits to drinking excessively and stopping his medication again'*. This time, he is referred to a psychiatric nurse. In the referral letter, the GP will say that he will be grateful if together they can find a way to help Gary *'sort out this apparently abnormal grief reaction'*.

Ah, good doctor. Define 'abnormal' for me. I'll wait.

Shades is back at the surgery the following month, on a Wednesday afternoon at the end of June, for his first meeting with the psychiatric nurse. In his notes he records first impressions of my brother: a *'small, slightly built 25-year-old man'* (his weight has dropped to just over nine stone) who presents as *'anxious and restless'*. He is *'neatly and appropriately dressed'* and his speech is *'normal in form'* but he has *'difficulty articulating his thoughts'*, thoughts that are *'dominated by feelings of loss and regret'*.

Gary tells him that his childhood was 'basically happy' but that he 'never really settled in at the school' and eventually, after several shop-floor jobs, he became an apprentice joiner. During this period, the late 80s and early 90s, his relationship with his father became 'a little strained' (*'where the bloody hell have ye been tae this time o' the morning?' 'Lee me alane – get tae fuck'*) but that they became 'more friendly' after he moved out of the family home to live in a flat near his parents' house.

'And I gather,' the nurse asks, glancing at the notes sent to him by the GP, 'you've not been coping too well since your dad died, Gary?'

'Eh, naw. It wiznae too bad for the couple o' months, wi' aw the funeral arrangements tae deal wi' and that, ken? But since then . . . it's jist been getting worse.' Shades goes on, telling him about how, after dad had got cancer, he'd moved back into the family home 'to help look after him, ken?' He talks about how dad had been improving but then, last April, he died very suddenly. 'Ah never really got a chance tae talk tae him properly. Jist keep thinking aboot that aw the time. Cannae stop it. Cannae sleep so Ah cannae.' He tells the psychiatrist about how his personality has changed. How he used to be 'outgoing' and 'sociable' but has become 'irritable' and 'isnae going oot much'.

Has withdrawn from social contact, the nurse will write.

'How are the rest of your family coping?'

'Jist . . . they jist seem to be getting oan wi' it, ken?'

'Are you able to talk about your feelings with them?'

'Naw. Naw. Linda's jist a wee lassie, so she is. John's away now, doon in London. Ah don't want tae go on tae ma maw aboot it. It'd jist upset her, ken?'

'So how are you coping?'

'Ah jist . . . Ah've been drinking a lot.'

The nurse notes that Gary is currently drinking '15–20 units on three or four days of the week. 60–80 units of alcohol a week.'

'Do you ever drink until you lose consciousness?'

'Aye, sometimes.'

'Why do you think you seem to be coping worse than the rest of your family?'

It comes out. 'Ah . . . Ah feel guilty, doketar. So Ah dae. Ah, Ah caused a lot o' havoc at hame, ye know? Just wi, when Ah wiz younger, wi' buzzing the glue and the partying an other hings. Dogging the school and aw that. Fighting wi' ma da aw the time.'

'Physically, you mean?'

'Aye. Sometimes. Aye.'

His face, looking up from the kitchen floor, beseeching.

'Ah just . . . we hud a lot o' unfinished business.'

'You and your father?'

'Aye.'

The psychiatric nurse's conclusions: Gary is 'clinically depressed'. He has 'chronic insomnia'. He appears to have 'rather bottled up his emotions' and, one year on from dad's death, 'his grief reaction has become pathological in its duration'. He is referred to a bereavement counsellor and prescribed the 'sedative antidepressant' Trazodone to help him sleep at night.

Shades comes out of the surgery and into the spring sunshine,

213

clutching his prescription as he turns right towards the pharmacy. The Pleasure Dome up above the old Co-op, where, just a few years earlier, the future had seemed endless and beautiful and strafed by green lasers.

Six weeks after his appointment with the psychiatric nurse, in the middle of September, Gary meets with the bereavement counsellor, who confirms the PN's findings. He gives him information leaflets on depression and anxiety and outlines an action plan: 1) to encourage the 'ventilation' of Gary's feelings, 2) to re-establish him on Prozac, and 3) to see him again in a few weeks' time. Shades fails to return for that appointment. Or for their next two scheduled meetings. Instead, he begins to try and deal with his unprocessed grief the same way I am.

We both start throwing ourselves into our 'work' . . .

Solid Gold Easy Listening

Christian Tattersfield and I fly to Munich on a Saturday morning in November, where we have three of our acts – Orbital, CJ Bolland and The Advent – performing at Tribal Gathering 1995, in a huge aircraft hangar on the outskirts of the city.

I'd met Tattersfield the year before. We're the same age, but he's been working at a major record company for four years and is, by some distance, sharper and more cynical than I am. London Records have given him his own label, Internal, and he's released albums by Orbital and a string of pop-dance hits, climaxing the previous summer with Whigfield's million-selling 'Saturday Night'. The success of the record gave Tattersfield the leeway to hire his own marketing person. Me. I'm earning thirty grand a year now, finally making more than my age in

214

money. I have a seemingly bottomless expense account and a company car. I have a flat in Notting Hill. Stephanie is still in Glasgow. She's five months pregnant and our relationship is fracturing, because I'm so caught up in this exciting new life. Because I'm spending the week in London living that life and the weekends in Glasgow living another kind. Because, well, because of stuff like this – flying to Munich to get out of my mind for twenty-four hours and calling the apocalypse of pills and coke and strong German beers and shots 'work'.

And it hadn't taken me long to realise that the real action at a record company doesn't reside in the marketing department, in among the rolled 60x40 posters and the glossy proofs of artwork. It lives further up the building, amongst the sacks of demo tapes and the racks of gleaming hi-fi equipment in the A&R department on the third floor. These guys have power, cachet. They roll in at lunchtime. They get huge salaries, bonuses and percentage points on records. A few months into the job, I've decided I need to sign a hit record, to catapult myself out of the world of barcodes and checking label copy and making sure some posters go up near the band manager's house, and up onto the third floor. This was where you'd hear rudimentary versions of songs blasting out of offices that, just a few weeks or months later, were suddenly in the charts. Cast, The Longpigs, Audioweb, Gene, Mansun, Elastica – I hear all these bands blaring out of offices in demo form in the months after I join the company. All of them are the subject of mad A&R scrambles. Because guitar-band fever is rolling across the country in the wake of an act not totally dissimilar to some of those who I ploughed the indie circuit with just a few years earlier. There's a crucial difference this time though: forget holding his shirt out and pretending to have tiny breasts while whining,

'*Ooooh, Ah'm Morrissey, pump me daft,*' this is a Manchester band that Shades, and millions more like him, will *love*.

Early the next day, Sunday, running on very little sleep, we fly back to London. On the cab ride in from Heathrow, we're listening to the chart rundown on Radio 1. As we come along the flyover of the Great West Road towards Hammersmith – the *Bladerunner* stretch, illuminated signage towering over us: Audi, Porsche, that bubbling Lucozade bottle forever emptying into its glass, replacing '*lost energy*', oh, man, if only it were that simple – Mark Goodier says 'and this week's highest new entry, straight in at number two, "Wonderwall" by Oasis . . .'

'Ha!' Tattersfield laughs, delighted. 'The filthy Mancunian animals get done up the shitter by Cowell's bricklayers. Too good.'

It's a reference to warbling meat puppets Robson and Jerome, the housewives' choice signed by Simon Cowell over at BMG, who have just succeeded in keeping Oasis off the number one spot. Tattersfield is heading home, but the cab drops me first, at Earl's Court, for the second night of Oasis's two-night stint there. 'Make sure you mention the bricklayers at the aftershow,' he says as I get out and he drives away, laughing his head off.

Creation have gone to town.

I take in the gigantic vertical-strip banners flanking the venue, illuminated by Klieg lights, towering over the 20,000 people making their way inside: Noel on the left, Liam on the right, a band taking their place at the very centre of the culture. Inside there's Tony Crean, Barrett and Kelly, Paolo Hewitt, Sean Rowley. Fucking *Goldie* is here. I drop an E. The band go straight into 'Acquiesce' and it feels like you're at the heart of something. Then the after-party. And then the party after that.

And then and then and then. Glossy rectangles of paper and Hooch and squat brown bottles getting shoved under your nose and your skull flaring out like a match head and my new, purple Soho House membership card scrubbing powder through a fifty-pound note and, finally, somewhere in the early hours of the Monday morning, bed.

The Player

Shot from behind, the camera following on the dolly, Shades comes striding through the coastal breeze of Ayr and up the broad sandstone steps, his shoulders working, confident and purposeful, the tiny silver eagle on the back right-hand pocket of his Armani jeans, the 'GA' in its talons, catching the light, glinting in the dusk. He's here on business. A nod to the security guys – no search, they know him – and he strolls on into the noise pounding out of the building, the structure itself seeming to rear up on its foundations, as though its Edwardian gentility is offended by what is taking place within, boiling in its insides, beneath its turrets and balustrades.

By the beginning of the 90s, the gigs had tailed off and things were looking bleak for Ayr Pavilion, where I thrilled to Charlie Harper all those years ago. And then unlikely saviours arrive – the likes of The Prodigy, Ultrasonic, DyeWitness, Human Resource, Ramirez. Hanger 13 launches in March 1993 and quickly becomes one of Scotland's premier rave venues. Clubbers travel down from as far afield as Glasgow, Falkirk, Livingston and Edinburgh to lose themselves in the strobe-lit clouds of dry ice, lasers strafing the murk, the squat towers of the bassbins, black as crows, squelching, all of it fuelled by a cascade of ecstasy. It feels like heaven. It feels like the future.

217

Shades, an ambassador of the future, moves through all of this, along the edge of the dancefloor where hundreds are losing themselves to Trevor Reilly on the decks, and towards the bar at the opposite end. He returns shouts, nods, hellos and handshakes with heavy-ringed paws. Embraces and kisses from girls. This is a *player*.

'Shades! Awright, wee boy?'

'Awright, bud?'

'Hey, can ye—'

'Aye, aye – gies a minute, hen.'

'Shadesy-boy!'

'Whit's happening, ma man?'

The player takes his place at the bar with his boys and tilts the long-necked bottle of Bud to his lips. His hand slides into his back pocket, snug under that eagle. The big package has been divided into smaller ones. The conversations yelled into ears surrounded by damp hair in dark corners – *There ye go, doll. Aye, cheers. Sort us oot later. Naw. Mitsubishis. Ye already owe us fur four. Huvin' a good time? The state o' him. Nae bother, wee man. Aye, plenty. Awright, wee sacks? Smoke ma dobber.*

The business gets done. The crowd heaves, their hands in the air, clapping and whooping as another breakdown drops. His own pill is kicking in now as he moves in front of the speaker stack, head bobbing side to side, fingers pointing, the neck of his Bud in his left hand, the snare starting the long fill that will bring the bassline back in.

Ooommffff.

It drops and the place goes mad: sweat spraying through white light bursts. He catches moments in Polaroid flashes – a boy pouring a bottle of water over his head in the middle of the scrum, cheeks blown out like a swimmer finishing, exploding through the surface. A girl with

218

long, curly hair plastered to her face with sweat, eyes closed, her movements flickering crazily in the stop-start of the strobes. The chopping hands of the dancers on the balcony, performing karate on their invisible enemies. Shades throws his head back as he raises his own hands and looks up, following the skeins of steam rising from the dancers, all the way up to the great roof, bolted into place the year *Titanic* sailed, sitting over all of this as impartially as it once looked down upon the gently waltzing Edwardian couples.

And then, in April 1994, eighteen-year-old John Nisbet from New Cumnock collapses on this very dancefloor and dies after taking one and a half pills. The following month Andrew Dick, nineteen, from Glasgow, dies in a similar incident. In August Andrew Stoddart, twenty, from Lanarkshire, also falls into a coma and dies after taking ecstasy at the club.

It is now what the papers are calling a 'string' of deaths. Following a fatal accident inquiry in Glasgow, Sheriff Neil Gow, QC, warns that 'a dance with ecstasy is a dance with death'. A few months later, in November, four hundred miles south, an Essex teenager called Leah Betts dies after taking ecstasy and drinking seven litres of water in ninety minutes. For the tabloids her death becomes a rallying point, and the pressure increases on police forces across the country to do something about the 'deadly new leisure drug'.

Up in Glasgow, Strathclyde Police begin formulating plans for a massive crackdown on Scotland's drug trade. They will use the same symbol that glints on the back pocket of my brother's Armani jeans, catching on the Hanger 13 lights as he moves to the whump of the bass.

Operation Eagle launches later that year.

★   ★   ★

A few days after the Oasis show, I'm drinking in the Groucho Club, at the crowded downstairs bar, when someone says, 'John, you know Joe, right?' I turn to shake hands and find myself looking into the deep hazelnut eyes of Joe Strummer. 'All right?' Strummer says. 'What you drinking, mate?' He's all in black – jeans, T-shirt and suit jacket – and, mercifully, he doesn't seem to remember the white leather biker's jacket from fourteen years earlier. Besides, that kid is long gone. He's been replaced by a hip, swaggering twentysomething sophisticate who casually asks for a Seabreeze and tells the barman to put it all on his tab. Who makes easy small talk about Black Grape and Glastonbury and makes it very clear he no longer gives a solitary fuck about the whereabouts of Mick Jones. Who, four or five drinks in, with effortless grace and charm, looks into those hazelnut eyes and says, 'Hey, Joe – do you fancy a nose up?' And, moments later, in the downstairs cubicle, with me chopping the powder with the credit card, gibbering away about whatever, I look up to see the poised nostrils of Strummer lowering towards me like the barrels of a shotgun as I pass up the rolled fifty. As tradition dictates, Joe immediately re-rolls the note, tighter.

We're at the bar a few hours, many Seabreezes and several trips to the cubicle later, when I finally get it out. 'Y-you changed my life.' Strummer, waiting to get served, just nods and gently, sympathetically, squeezes my forearm. 'Fuck,' I say. 'You must be sick to death of hearing that.'

'Shit, John,' he says. 'Who'd get sick of hearing that?'

The Groucho shuts, and Joe and I take a cab around to Farringdon, where the Heavenly guys have a club night running at the Jazz Bistro. The only analogous experience to walking into a Heavenly Records night with Joe Strummer might be strolling into church of a Sunday morning hand in hand with Jesus Christ. People line up to buy Strummer drinks, and the night breaks apart into the usual cascade of drinking and cheeky halves and passed wraps and your head flaring up here and there as a squat brown bottle is unexpectedly jammed under your nose – *Happy Birthday, Danny!* – and plasticfacecarntsmilewhiteout.

At one point, late in the night, I become aware that I've lost Joe. He'd been telling me earlier that he'd missed the last train home – he'd recently moved to Basingstoke (?!) – and I'd offered him a bed at our flat in Notting Hill. Someone says he's in the toilet. I go in to find the bathroom empty, but the cubicle occupied. 'Joe?' I rap on the door. 'Joe? Are you OK, man?' Muffled shouting. I knock some more. Suddenly the door flies open and Strummer charges out shouting, 'OK! OK! JESUS CHRIST!' I don't know that he sees me. He just strides straight out into the club, then through the club, and out the front door onto Farringdon Road. I follow, shouting after him, 'Joe! Joe!' But no, he's not stopping, just striding off into the night, talking to himself, pointing at the sky.

Then he's gone.

I wind up at a party for the promoter Harvey Goldsmith, at the Hanover Grand, just off Regent Street. The musical entertainment is an easy-listening outfit called The Mike Flowers Pops. The musicians sit on stools – very much Ronnie Hazlehurst's TV orchestra circa 1978 – and Mike himself conducts them. He wears a sky-blue suit and a blond wig cut in a vicious bowl, occasionally turning around to throw a shit-eating grin at the audience as they work through a slick, bossa nova–ish take on classics from the 60s and 70s, everything from my parents' beloved 'The Age Of Aquarius' to 'Light My Fire'.

I watch three or four songs before I wander off in search of diversion and bump into my friend Liam, who works for Harvey and is very much a man-about-town. It turns out that he booked Mike Flowers for the party. Hunkered over a gram in the bathroom, Liam talks knowledgably about London's emergent lounge-core scene, about clubs like Indigo and Blow Up and DJs like The Karminsky Experience. But really, I couldn't give a shit. None of this sounds like it'll produce a hit record and I need a hit record like I need the line he's taking forever racking out. 'Yeah, yeah,' I say. 'Great.'

Late the next morning, hungover after just a few hours' sleep, I wander into London Records, where I bump into my colleague Nick Raphael on the way up the stairs. Like me, Raphael had started in marketing before making the leap to A&R. Always on, forever hustling, he asks me, 'What did you get up to last night? See any gigs?'

'Saw this band in Mayfair — Mike Flowers Pops.'

'Unsigned?'

'I should think so.'

'Any hits?' The eternal A&R question.

'Nah. All covers.'

'Fuck them,' Raphael says.

And that's that.

Somewhat Inarticulate

After weeks of missed appointments and non-contact, Gary suddenly gets back in touch with the psychiatric nurse, requesting a new appointment.

He sees him on 16 November, a few days after what would have been dad's seventieth birthday. He asks Gary what has brought him back.

'Aye. Eh, ma uncle died.' (Our uncle, John Murray – cancer.) 'It's made me . . . eh, Ah've just started thinking about ma dad again. Aw the time. It wid huv been his birthday the other day, so it wid.'

The nurse checks his notes. 'Has the Prozac helped at all?'

'Naw. Ah mean, Ah stopped taking it. Made us feel no right, so it did. Aw funny. Couldnae sleep, so Ah couldnae.'

'Yes, but you need to keep taking it in order to–'

'Naw.' Gary's flat refusal. Wants what he wants. Or doesn't want.

'And how have you been sleeping since you stopped?'

'No much better. Cannae sleep at aw unless Ah've hud a lot tae drink, ken?'

The nurse notes that Gary says he 'wishes to talk through his feelings' but that it then becomes 'difficult' for him to do so. *'Somewhat inarticulate.'* He is prescribed Prothiaden – the brand name for dosulepin, at the time the most frequently prescribed antidepressant in the UK – and a follow-up appointment is scheduled. But again, Gary fails to show up. The psychiatric nurse writes to his GP: 'I will not be sending Gary any further appointments in the meantime.'

But, soon after, Gary calls out of the blue, requesting to be seen again by the nurse. An appointment is arranged, but once again Gary – increasingly the kind of erratic, selfish patient that bedevils the NHS – fails to show up. Finally, the nurse visits Gary at home, at 143 Livingstone Terrace, where Gary and mum are still living together. Gary initially blames his non-appearance at the previous appointments on 'panic attacks' and a 'phobia about hospitals', but he soon admits to suffering from 'lapses of memory'. The reason for these lapses quickly become apparent when he's asked (and, from the honesty of his answers, mum is clearly not present at this meeting) how his drinking is now.

'Ach, bad so it is. No every day, but maybe four or five days a week.'

'How much are you drinking on these days, Gary?'

'Maybe a bottle o' vodka? Or twelve cans o' lager?' The scratch of the medic's pen across the paper, the tick of the clock above the fireplace. Gary's keys and loose change on the mantelpiece that dad built.

'Why do you think you're drinking so much?' The psychiatric nurse writes in his notes: *currently 150–250 plus units alcohol per week. Disturbed sleep pattern. Disturbed dietary intake. Poor concentration. Flat affect. Lacking in volition.*

'Jist tae, ken, block oot ma feelings. Tae stop maself thinking. Ah feel worse when Ah'm sober. Keep huvin' panic attacks an that. Cannae sleep.'

'Are you using any medication?'

'Aye, Temazepam sometimes.'

'On prescription?' The puzzled look at the notes, checking.

'Naw, jist aff a mate, ken?' The guilty shuffling, looking at the floor.

'I see. Is there any other illicit drug use?'

'Well, aye . . . weed. And . . .' The shuffling increasing, the eyes darting, checking the corners as he lowers his voice. 'Heroin, sometimes. Jist a wee bit. Jist smoking it, ken?'

There is a note right next to this admission in his file, scrawled in the margin in upper case.

'NOT KNOWN TO MOTHER.'

These words have, of course, a dual resonance.

I Am Become Death

A few days after the night of Strummer, my alarm clock wakes me promptly at 8.30 in the flat in Notting Hill, with the Chris Evans breakfast show on Radio 1. I'm yawning and scratching as, along with eighteen million other listeners, I find myself listening to 'Wonderwall'. Except not. It's the song, yes, but it sounds pre-Beatles, like it's been beamed through wires from 1962. The style of it is oddly familiar. Bossa nova-ish. The kind of record my dad might have had. The track ends and Evans says, 'Well, we've found Noel Gallagher out now, right? That was the *original* version of "Wonderwall" by The Mike Flowers Pops and I'm going to be playing that every single morning this week.' A second or two goes by before I *explode* out of bed and scrabble for my address book and the phone. I'm shaking as I dial the number, already thinking of Raphael, who forgets nothing, in the A&R meeting . . .

'Yeah, Niven saw them the other night! Clown said there were no hits!'

'Liam? You've got to introduce me to Mike Flowers. Now. This morning.'

A few hours later, Mike and I meet for lunch in a French bistro near his home in Battersea. Red wine and cassoulet. He's in his mid-thirties, a graduate of Chelsea Art School, with a gentle Liverpool accent, and his real name is Mike Roberts.

Unwigged, Mike turns out to be very smart: dry, sharp and nicely cynical, with a keen musical intelligence. We offer him £25,000 for the rights to the single with an option for an album. No fool he – with other labels hammering at the door and very aware that Chris Evans playing your record every day of the week to, in Tattersfield's words, 'eighteen million disgraceful toerags' equates to a guaranteed Top 10 single – Mike gets £50,000 out of us and grants no album option. We'll have to negotiate that down the road, which could put us on the back foot if the single really does some business. It is mid-November now. We have four weeks to do artwork, cobble together some B-sides, manufacture, launch a poster campaign, make a video and try and have the Christmas number one. It's all a bit like Band Aid, had Band Aid solely been for the benefit of a room full of rich, coked-up white men. Having the Christmas number one quickly becomes a fierce matter of pride for London Records as we did it the year before with East 17's 'Stay Another Day'. Demand for Mike's version is already high and building every day. According to the sales force, despite strong ongoing sales for Michael Jackson's dismal planet-hugging 'Earth Song', we are looking like we will *just* take the number one spot come Christmas week.

Lots of people at the label are starting to place bets on the record doing just this. Chairman Tracy Bennett sends someone over to Ladbrokes in Hammersmith to stick a few grand on at something like 30–1. Like Oppenheimer, I become so wrapped up in the 'how-do-we-do-this?' that I fly right by the question of 'should-we-be-doing-this?' Fuelled by cocaine, greed and hubris, in a few short years I have gone from wondering how Maurice Deebank from Felt got his acoustic guitar sound to screaming at the production department because the inserts for the cassette format of the novelty record I've signed might not be ready in time to meet Our Price's order. Sony, meanwhile, are throwing everything at trying to keep Jackson at number one for a fourth week. He's already seen off The Bricklayers, Boyzone, Oasis themselves and *The fucking Beatles*. Tattersfield and I gee the company up, urging everyone – marketing, radio and TV promotions, the press office – to work harder, to leave no stone unturned, to think of the contest in David and Goliath terms. Come Christmas week it is extremely tight on the midweeks – we are number one on the Tuesday and then Jackson takes us out on Wednesday and then it's back to us on Thursday. 'Everyone's got the Jackson record,' the sales force tells us. 'We'll be the big sales gainer on Saturday . . .'

Christmas Eve, Sunday, 24 December 1995, rolls around.

I'm back up from London for the holidays, hunched by the radio in the kitchen of the flat in the West End of Glasgow. It's just before 7pm when Goodier finally gets to it. 'And, at number two . . .'

I am due a bonus of ten grand for a number one record. I am thinking I might be able to double my, already generous, salary. I am thinking about new offices, up on the top floor, job offers from other labels. Upgrading the company car . . .

227

Tracy stands to win a couple of hundred grand. Not a life-changing sum for the man who signed Bananarama, Fine Young Cannibals, East 17 and – very soon – All Saints, but it'd certainly slim down his tab at the Groucho for a bit. As Goodier's ludicrous dramatic pause goes on for what feels like eternity, I am praying to hear the words, 'down, after three weeks at number one', praying to hear the over-blown, ominous synth, the tinkling piano trills and then Jackson plaintively asking us 'what about sunrise?' *Yeah, what about it, you fucker?* And then Goodier says, 'This week's highest new entry . . .'

Oh no. Please no.

The gently stabbing brass, the unwinding string section and Mike's fruity baritone singing the opening words of 'Wonderwall'. I start screaming and cursing and smacking the table, doubling over with rage as I bellow, *'FUCK YOU, FUCK!'* Stephanie, nearly seven months pregnant now, runs in. 'What the hell is the matter with you?'

Karma goes about its business, ensuring that I feel the sharp pain of Noel Gallagher, just the month before, in the dressing room at Earl's Court, when Goodier announced the number two record and he too heard the dread words 'this week's highest new entry . . .'

Three weeks later, in the middle of all this, our son Robin is born, five weeks premature, the size of a bag of sugar, but full of life, full of fight. The midwife holds the screaming haunch of meat up to me in the delivery room. He only has one eye open and we make direct eye contact. One real thing in the midst of all this froth and distraction, of the midweeks and marketing spends and guest lists. However, in the interest of full disclosure, and mindful of the guys lurking with rubber pipe and rolled telephone book, at the time it feels the other way around to me.

Ongoing Mental State

The community psychiatric nurse calls on Gary again early in the new year of 1996, as arranged. But he is not at home. He leaves a note, asking Gary to call him to arrange yet another appointment.

Reading Gary's medical records today, a quarter of a century later, I am struck by the kindness and patience of the medics. The phone-book-thick file on my desk records dozens of missed appointments, broken arrangements and medication strategies agreed upon then unilaterally abandoned by Gary.

I am amazed by the gentle, caring persistence of the healthcare professionals with people whose lifestyles – the Valium, the cannabis, the heroin, the 250-plus units of alcohol every week – make it impossible for them to adhere to even the simplest plans. Another appointment is made and then falls through too. (Panic attack/phobia/memory lapse/whatever.)

It is February 1996 when they finally sit down together again, once more in the living room at mum's house. After this consultation the nurse writes a short note to Gary's GP. *'He continues to present with depressive symptoms which appear to be related to the multiple bereavements within his family. He denies any illicit drug use'* (this making me think that mum must have been present this time) *'though he continues to use alcohol with its primary function being as an hypnotic. With this in mind, perhaps you would consider recommencing him on his previous antidepressant medication, which I believe was Prothiaden, which Mr Niven discontinued of his own volition. I have reinforced the need to adhere to a prescribed medication regime with Mr Niven and I have arranged to see him again at home in two weeks' time to further assess his ongoing mental state.'*

Unsurprisingly, this appointment does not happen.

There are no further medical records for Gary for nearly two years. He slips off the radar. Stops trying to get whatever help he's been trying to get.

The next entry is another note from the same psychiatric nurse, again to Gary's GP. It was written on 15 October 1997. It is even shorter, consisting of a single sentence.

'*I am discharging Gary from my case load as I believe he's currently in prison.*'

Praxis

London Records is not a gentle, nurturing environment. What the company thrives on, and excels at, is Big Hit Singles. And the beast requires constant feeding.

By February, around the time I am sauntering back into the office following paternity leave, the fevered race for the Christmas number one is already a distant memory and it is very much a case of 'what-have-you-done-for-me-lately?' What we *should* have done with Mike was to record a live album and bang it out in January, into a soft chart and straight off the back of a huge hit single. (Despite missing the number one slot, his version of 'Wonderwall' still sold half a million copies.) But, with no album option, we are over a barrel. Which means acceding to Mike's plans: recording with a full orchestra at Livingston Studios at considerable expense. Meanwhile we scramble to get a follow-up single out. London MD Colin Bell thinks we should have Mike do something incongruously punk rock – 'Anarchy In The UK' or 'White Riot'. I think this is a terrible idea.

I'm championing his flamboyant take on 'The "In" Crowd', which I argue has just the right level of knowing postmodernism, a cheeky nod to Mike's sudden elevation to fame and its undoubtedly transient nature. I am told in no uncertain terms to forget all this shite and come back with a proper hit single. Colin and I have endless screaming matches and, as a compromise, we end up going with 'Light My Fire', a staple of Mike's live set. We are rewarded with another Top 40 smash.

It goes straight in at number thirty-nine. Then vanishes.

An interesting thing begins to happen. I am already familiar with the expression 'success has a thousand fathers – failure is an orphan', but, like Goldman's 'screenplays are structure', it is a phrase I have so far only understood in the conceptual, the abstract. I begin to get a valuable lesson in *praxis*.

When we signed Mike and we (record executives always use the royal 'we' when talking about their acts) were all over the radio in the headlong rush for the Christmas number-one spot, the project was very much known around the company as 'Tattersfield's new signing'. As the tortured process of recording the album and choosing a follow-up single began to unfold, Mike became 'Tattersfield and Niven's signing'. By the time we've had a single go in at thirty-nine with an anchor and we've spent three months and hundreds of thousands of pounds recording the album, it has mysteriously very much become simply 'Niven's signing'.

Finally, after Mike has overdubbed the last clavinet, xylophone and bassoon parts, after he's nailed every harmony and cymbal crash, we release the album *A Groovy Place* in June 1996, in a clean white sleeve showing Mike lounging confidently in a huge black leather armchair.

We sell three thousand copies.

Game over.

See you later, Sooty.

Failure is an orphan, and here I was, running the J. Niven Home for Hitless Acts. Tattersfield sashays through the carnage untouched. Like the hitman Leon, bullets slide off him. And there's me, writhing and spasming in a hail of lead: Jimmy Caan at the tollbooth in *The Godfather*, Beatty and Dunaway in the car in *Bonnie and Clyde*, Peter Weller in front of Clarence's gang in *Robocop*.

Where, I keep asking myself, did those other 497,000 people who bought the single go? Well, it transpires that relying on the repeat business of a few hundred thousand drunken office workers who bought a mad cover version of an Oasis song as a kind of funny Christmas present six months ago is no way to build an actual fanbase.

Who knew?

The Mule

March 29, 1996. It is a night I often picture him on.

Gary is living in a flat again, in one of the Orlit houses on Woodlands Avenue, near Basil's old place, opposite the playing fields and the dug track, just a ten-minute walk from the house that is no longer mum and dad's, that is now just mum's house.

It's a Friday night and Ayrshire is slipping into her party clothes, with kids in the houses in the surrounding streets all doing what Shades is doing now: coming into the bedroom fresh from the shower, buttoning shirts over damp chests, pulling up designer jeans, with Pete Tong's show pumping from the radio. Shades dabs a final splash of aftershave on (Polo Sport by Ralph Lauren) and gels his hair in the mirror. He lights a Club, takes a Bud Ice from the fridge – tin-foil tubs of Chinese leftovers and maw's Pyrex bowl with a wee bit of that beef stew she brought round – and paces the living room.

It's cold and blustery out, but at least it's still light, bars of sunshine in the watery sky. The clocks will go forward on Sunday, spring finally arriving. Easter next weekend. Just after 6.30 he hears the rumble of tyres, the squeak of the handbrake, and looks out the window to see a car pull up outside. Because, on a Friday night, in her party clothes,

233

Ayrshire has her party needs. It's Jock. The Boss. A few years older than Shades, Jock is a major player by 1996. Lost as I am at the time in the plans for a second Mike Flowers single, it will be Linda who fills me in, later, on what he's like, and what Shades is becoming like in proximity to him.

She'd been at a house party one night, a very late-night affair, with everyone bent out of shape, dropping cans, spilling drinks, a real chimp's tea party deal. Shades and Jock were both there, supplying party essentials. Everyone was smoking constantly – joints, fags – and Jock, Linda noticed out of the corner of her eye, started unobtrusively pocketing lighters as they did the rounds. Soon the refrains were becoming more and more frequent: 'anyone got a light?' or 'who's got my lighter?' Linda noticed that Jock was that bit more sober than everyone else. She noticed the quiet pleasure he seemed to be taking as the paralytic mob became more and more frustrated at this minor inconvenience. The gentle smirk on his face as someone else patted themselves down and searched their pockets for a few minutes before giving in and finally asking, 'Fuck sake! Who's got a light?' Later, his game complete, Linda saw him dump a dozen or so disposable lighters into a bowl in the hall, translucent purples and reds and greens, like day-glo sticks. It was a *piccolo* torture to be sure, but revealing. Control. Superiority. 'You got a sense he was taking everything in,' Linda said. Calculating. Devious.

Towards dawn, Linda was in the kitchen, making tea, when Gary came in. The two of them started laughing and joking around, shooting lines from films and TV shows at one another (all the Niven children: prodigious libraries of movie quotes) when, suddenly, Jock entered the room. Wordlessly his steely, beady gaze settled on

234

Shades, as if to say 'what are you doing in here, laughing and talking shite?' As if to say, 'this is not appropriate behaviour for a gangsta playa.' As if to say 'stop it.' And he did. Instantly. The moment Jock entered, Gary's personality changed entirely as he donned his other persona – the gruff, monosyllabic hardman – and said goodbye to Linda. He followed Jock out of the room, then out of the flat, then off into the night, to wherever what they supplied was needed at that hour of the morning.

Shades takes a last, hurried sip of the Bud Ice, grabs his Stone Island parka and runs out to the car. They do the basics on the drive from Irvine over to Ayr, Jock at the wheel, the countryside around them just beginning to warm up, the earliest leaves on the trees between the bypass and the sea. There are some nerves jangling in the car, underneath the tunes coming from the cassette player, but not too much. They're pros. Not their first rodeo. Here on business. They park the car on the street in the estate in Ayr just after 7pm and come walking into the house of this girl they know. The moment they stroll in the front door, the plan changes.

Everything changes.

Instead of what they were expecting to find – tunes playing, bottles of beer being popped open, lines being chopped out, shouts of 'awright, boys!' and 'here we go!' – they are confronted by several officers from Strathclyde Police, who have already been there for some time, executing a search warrant.

Operation Eagle.

Shades and Jock are cautioned and then they are searched.

In his inside coat pocket Jock has £1,775 in notes. ('Ma savings,' he tells the officer.) In the rear pocket of his jeans, he has another

£200. In the front pocket he has £68.50, his walking-around money. He also has two uncashed Giros. Income Support cheques.

Shades has no money to speak of. What he does have is a plastic bag. Which, in turn, contains five smaller plastic bags, each containing around fifty ecstasy tablets: a total of two hundred and twenty-five pills. What went through his mind at this moment, as he was searched, knowing what he had in his pocket? As someone in the game he'd have known a bit about quantities and sentencing, about possession versus intent to supply, about Category A drugs v. Category B. And he'd certainly have known that, if things went south in the next few minutes, he'd be facing trial in Ayrshire, where all those kids had died in the last couple of years, just along the road at Hanger 13, after taking the very same drug that he has on him now in the hundreds. They are both arrested and charged with attempting to supply a Class A drug under the Misuse of Drugs Act 1971.

Except that, as far as Shades and Jock are concerned, there will be no 'they'. There will only be 'he'. Attempting to take the bullet, Shades pleads guilty right away, claiming that Jock had nothing to do with the drugs. In his turn, Jock attempts the defence that all the cash he has on him simply represented his own savings, which it was his right to do with as he pleased. His argument is undercut by the fact that he also has on him a list of names and phone numbers, very much like a client list, and that someone receiving those Income Support cheques is unlikely to have been able to save up over £2,000. The dynamic between Shades and Jock is clear enough to the police. At the trial, one of the arresting officers will sum up their relationship for the judge like this: 'It is common practice in the illicit drug trade to employ a mule to carry the drugs, someone who would take the risk of being found in possession while the dealer and others involved in the supplying would thereby be distanced.'

Shades – the mule.

And it is clear from the get-go that it is not him the police are after. He is offered a deal: tell us that Jock is the real dealer and you can walk away from all of this. No sale. Gary will not bend, will not buckle. Wee Shades? A grass? No way. He insists on his own guilt and Jock's innocence. Why? Out of a misguided west coast of Scotland small-time gangster interpretation of the rules of omertà? The idea of being a 'stand-up guy' who doesn't 'rat' on his friends? Probably. It's right there in the job description – the mule takes the hit. Because he's scared of Jock? That's surely in there too. But there's something else . . .

Shades had been well-chosen for his role. The wee boy who would throw the stones through the window; who would hurl the kid's shoes into the pond because the bigger boys dared him to do it; who would march at the head of the lunatics, their gleeful mascot. Not the biggest, the strongest or the hardest, but the one who was willing to go further than most of the others would, who was desperate to prove himself, to prove the value he hadn't been able to show at school or at home. Here was his chance to shine, to take the lead role in the drama.

'I did it,' he tells them. 'It was all me.'

Linda gets the call later on that night, from Jock's younger sister, telling her that Gary is being held at Kilmarnock Police Station. Frustrated, gunning for a bigger target, the police are refusing to accept his guilty plea and they will both be going to trial. Fortuitously, Linda's boyfriend Jim, the same Jim who had been threatened by Shades with a handgun that New Year a few years back, is now a trainee criminal lawyer, at the firm who end up representing Gary. Linda calls

Livingstone Terrace in the early hours of Saturday morning, the phone ringing on the hall table.

Mum coming down the stairs, already terrified by the call at this hour, the thought, *whit's that boy done now?* probably bubbling away. Her tremulous, suspicious 'Hello?'

'Mum?'

'Linda? Whit is—'

'Mum, you need to sit down.'

There aren't too many ways to phrase it: Gary has been arrested for dealing ecstasy and is very likely looking at a prison sentence. In the short hallway in Livingstone Terrace, mum clutches the telephone as she feels the breath being punched out of her, as she feels her legs giving way. She sits down on the landing at the bottom of the stairs – where the echo was good – and she breaks down. The sum of all fears:

Whit goes on in that boy's head?

Start a fight in an empty house, so he would.

Bad wee stick.

End up in the Bar-L.

Gary is released on police bail. The case will take a long time, over a year, to come to trial. In the meantime, he resumes his old ways. With gusto. Like his elder brother down in London, his lust for hedonism is fierce and will not desert him in the dark days of 1996/97. Indeed, Shades runs to engage life at its very core.

There's a few weans running aboot this toon wi' ma face . . .

The trial takes place at Kilmarnock Sheriff Court in the summer of 1997. Gary – the mule to the end – still claims it was all him. Jock

238

has fought on, determined to prove his innocence, to prove that he just happened to have his life savings of two thousand pounds – the two thousand pounds he carefully harvested from his benefits – on him, along with a long list of his friends' names and phone numbers, when he had been hanging out with his friend Gary, who just happened to have a couple of hundred Es on him when they walked into that house on a Friday night.

Jock gets five years.

And then the prosecution decides that they will now accept the guilty plea Shades had entered all along. The early guilty plea, their scheme to get Jock off, accidentally works in Gary's favour: the judge only sentences him to three years.

Only.

Mum doesn't go out much any more. Can't face the neighbours. She doesn't take her daily walk round to the shops at Caldon Road for the papers – her *Daily Record*, her *Irvine Herald* – for fear of what she might read in them about her son. She shuffles around the house where she raised a family, where she now lives alone, her husband dead, her daughter in Glasgow, one son in London and another in jail. At night she lies awake in bed and hears dad's dying words coming back to her – '*Look after the three of them.*'

On the first night Gary spends in prison, mum calls me broken with grief, looking for comfort as she keeps picturing her wee boy trying to sleep on his bunk, pulling the thin woollen blanket up under his chin in the cell deep in the bowels of that hellish jail. I do not remember this phone call at all – I would have been drunk and, most likely, coked-up – but, many years later, mum will tell me that I was distant, hurried, uninterested, dismissive. That we had people

239

over for dinner and I basically said, 'He'll be fine,' and went back to the guests, passing her over to Stephanie.

I look at that guy skulking in the line-up, lounging against the wall, squinting at the glass of the two-way mirror, and I think – *who are you?*

The Bar-L

I keep a photograph of my brother's football team in my desk drawer. It was taken in 1998. He is sitting on the far end of a bench, his hands clasped in front of him, three other players to his right, three more behind him. All the others wear shorts with navy and light blue striped jerseys, while Gary is in a grey top and with red tracksuit bottoms and thick gloves: the uniform of the goalkeeper. They are all smiling for the camera, and, at first glance, it looks like the standard team photo of any amateur seven-a-side mob, perhaps quietly pleased with themselves following a hard-fought victory after work on a Friday night. Ready to hit the showers and then the pub. Then you look closer, and you see the barbed wire topping the white wall in the distance, the wall with the number '2' sinisterly stamped on it in an authoritarian typeface. You see that the asphalt stretching away behind them is gradually revealing itself to be a yard, rather than a pitch.

HMP Barlinnie, Scotland's largest prison, is in Riddrie, to the north-east of Glasgow. It opened its doors in 1882 and is designed for punishment. Maximum grimness. Its blackened sandstone walls have contained Jimmy Boyle, Paul Ferris, Peter Manuel and Ali al-Megrahi, the man convicted of the Lockerbie bombing. Designed to accommodate around 1,000 inmates, by the late 90s it is routinely filled far, far

240

beyond this capacity. The practice of 'slopping out', of using in-cell buckets as toilets, persists in 1997, the year Shades arrives, the same year that a Scottish Prisons Inspectorate report describes the jail as 'a national disgrace'. Eight prisoners kill themselves during Gary's time there.

Mum makes the ninety-mile round trip to visit as often as she is allowed. She dresses in her best clothes and gets a lift up from Gary's friend, Craig. They get out of the car in the visitor car park, the monolithic block of the prison filling the sky ahead of mum, seeming to swallow her up with every step towards it. Once inside she will sit in a waiting room with the other visitors: some teenagers, some pensioners, but mostly people like her – *mothers*. The only ones who still have skin in the game at this point. She is searched for contraband – drugs, weapons – and then finally shown into the visiting area, where she will sit waiting for Gary to be brought out, trying, with her clothes, with her make-up, with all the force of her being, to project her goodness and decency, to project that she – and by extension her son – is not meant to be here. That he is a good boy who took a bad turn. That he was led astray. My wee mum, who thought her life was like a Hollywood film, with its cars and its bought house and the wine in its paper collar and setting the dining table on a Friday night for when her husband got home from the golf club.

All of it – blown away in a few short years.

Pinned

I visit him only once. *I'm busy. I'm a player.*

I fly up, hire a car at Glasgow Airport, and drive us – me and mum – out to Barlinnie. We go through a process that is, if not now routine

241

– it will never feel routine to her – at least familiar. We are paper-worked and frisked and badged and told the rules and regs and finally led into the visiting room, with its fluorescent tubes, its stale carpets, its vending machines, school chairs and chipped Formica tables. And this is the PR end of the prison, its best face. You sense the great machinery of incarceration contained just behind this curtain, the terrible weight of it. The prison guards stand silent around the room, looking straight ahead, like Beefeaters at the Tower. For me the experience is at once surreal and alien while not being completely unmediated. Because movies and literature have prepared me for it: the scene in *Goodfellas*, the barely glimpsed two-frames moment as the camera moves across the hellscape of the visiting room: the huge, bald con getting the hurried blowjob, nervously yet menacingly glancing around as he pushes down on the woman's head bobbing beneath the table. Or John Self in *Money*, visiting Alec in prison, in a room just like this one, *'a 60s coffee bar left to rot, windowless with bare-filament strip lighting and its heart-attack flicker'*, where Self comes to the realisation that *'I cannot put real distance between myself and prison. I can only put money there. It's in the blood, the blood.'*

Finally, Gary is led in and slides down across from us, grinning weakly. My first thought is – *Jesus Christ*.

His eyes are pinned, the pupils the size of the hole in the point of a hypodermic, his face sallow, almost the yellow of a legal pad.

'Awright, maw? John. Ye jist up, aye?'

His speech is creamy, spacey, slurred. I risk a sideways look at mum, to see if she is seeing and hearing the same things I am. If she is, she is choosing to ignore them. For she is already talking, filling him in on family comings and goings, news about Linda, about our cousins, about the dog, about life back home, in the world he has left behind. She talks on, seemingly unperturbed by his non-responses, as if she has decided to just have a nice wee chat with her son who has popped round to see her and get his washing done. As if she has decided to ignore the fact that Gary is smacked out of his gourd in prison. I do not know it, but I will see this exact mode of communication again, twelve years from now, in another institutional room, where the silent sentries are the graphite faces of machinery, where the background noises are the hiss and rasp of the ventilator, the footsteps of the nurses. I try for humour, teeing Gary up with some prison questions, clichés from the movies.

'Hey, Shades, on your first day in the dining hall, did you have to take out Mr Big with a sharpened tray or something, to stake your claim?'

'Naw, ye eat in your cell.'

'Bull queers in the showers?'

'Naw, John.'

We buy him sugary coffees and some chocolate bars that he keeps for later and, somehow, we get through the hour. On the way out, mum does not say a word, just keeps her gaze fixed straight ahead. The message is clear enough – *we will not be talking about this.* You have never felt relief as sharp, nor tasted air so sweet, or seen skies as endless and tropical, as when you step out of Barlinnie prison. The bleak suburb of Riddrie looks like Beverly Hills. We will not be talking about it, but, bull-headed as ever, I have to have a go. 'Is he always like that, mum?'

'Like what?'

'Well . . .'

243

'He's just tired, John.'

I look back at the place as we get in the rental car, thinking of him being led back through the cold passages, tiled when Victoria was on the throne, beneath the metal walkways with the nets strung across them to catch the jumpers, back to the 8x10 cell shared with three others, with his Twixes and Mars bars in his pockets, where he will spend most days being locked down for twenty-three hours, eating congealed food from a plastic tray, made by the lowest bidder and then microwaved half a mile away an hour earlier, where he will crouch over a bucket to defecate while his cellmates politely turn to face the wall. I think about all of this and I think something like – *fair enough, Shades.*

Shoot it up. Why not, pal?

Artiste and Repertoire

Back in the real world of A&R, after nearly twenty years, Joe Strummer is finally free from his contract with Sony and is looking for a new record deal.

Go! Discs recently relaunched Paul Weller's ice-cold solo career. I'm thinking something like, well, with the right record, you'd just scrub the name 'Weller' out on the marketing plan and write in 'Strummer'. But there's a problem. The tiny matter of having 'the right record'. Because, in all honesty, the demos aren't great. With all the force and belief of the convert, Joe has recently discovered the joys of ecstasy and dance music, and the first track on the CD is a number called 'Techno D-Day'. Its opening couplet tells us it was 'techno D–Day' on 'Omaha Beach' and it kind of makes my toes try to break themselves in the bending. More than the lyrical quibbles however, the melodies just aren't that compelling. It occurs to me that the problem might be that, unlike Weller, Strummer isn't a self-contained songwriting unit. Perhaps he needs a foil, an oppo, a tunesmith, a partner to bring the best out in him. I know far better than to suggest a rematching with Mick Jones, but maybe we could bring in a small pool of people to co-write, known Clash fans who'd jump at the chance to work with Joe. I'm thinking Roddy Frame, who we've recently signed to Independiente. James Dean Bradfield from the Manic Street Preachers. Maybe Andrew Innes from the Scream. Maybe the right cover version wouldn't be a bad idea? I sell this idea to myself very quickly: I see Joe's great comeback record going gold, then platinum. Triple platinum. Six times platinum. *Stanley* fucking *Road. Yeah, just scrub out 'Weller' on the marketing plan.* I see Joe accepting yet another award – a Brit, a Grammy – and tearfully thanking me one more time. Eager to tell him I've got the next phase of his career all worked out, I get his number from Norris. We've met socially a couple more times since the Groucho/Heavenly Social night, and Joe gracefully pretends to know me well. 'All right, John, how ya doing, mate? So, what did ya think of the demos then?'

I lay it all out for him: binning everything he's done so far. Starting again. Bradfield, Frame, Innes. An ominous cover version. World domination. There's a pause. In screenwriting terms you would call it 'a long beat'. Then the sound of the receiver being slammed down as, for the second time in my young life, an incensed Joe Strummer effectively tells me to get fucked.

'If you ever need anything . . .'

Gary is released from prison in the spring of 1999. I see him for the first time a few months later, on a work trip to Scotland for the T in the Park festival. ('Work.' Yeah, right.) I have braced myself for the encounter, fearing that he might have changed irreversibly, might have gone fully over to the other side, finally been transformed into a true hardman, into the Begbie he never really was. But no. It is

Shades, but Gary is still in there too, still with that nervous, shy energy – the eyes flitting around – masked by bravado, by the tendency to bluster too loudly.

'How ye doing?' I ask.

'Ach, fine, John, aye. Fine.'

But it transpires that his release began with a lie. He arrived back at mum's house early in the morning, clearly the worse for wear. It turned out that he'd been released a day earlier than he'd told mum he would, so he could ring-fence some time for a celebratory ecstasy frenzy over in Kilmarnock.

'Why?' I ask him.

'Ach, she'd just be wanting to keep me locked up here,' he gestured around, at the living room.

'Look, just try and not piss mum off, eh?'

'Aye. Awright. Gies peace, John.'

I sigh. 'Look, I gotta go. If you ever need anything, let me know, OK?' We embrace. Ralph Lauren, Polo Sport.

It will also transpire that the time Shades spent in prison has not been uneventful for him. Inside, he turned thirty. On the outside, he became a father, after a girlfriend called Nina gave birth to his son, Dale. Gary and Nina's relationship does not survive long after his release and he will only see Dale on an ad hoc basis, an arrangement terminated for good by Nina after 'Dale was in his care when there were drugs on the premises'. After this, mum is still allowed to see her grandson for a while until – apparently in contravention of their agreement – she allows Gary to see the boy one weekend when she is looking after him. This causes Nina to cut off all contact.

Gary will never see his son again.

I drive back to Glasgow, check into my room at the Malmaison, bang a couple of rails, and head down to the bar, where a scrum of my fellow A&R folk are gathering for T in the Park. There's Dan Keeling and Miles Leonard and Ferdy Unger-Hamilton and Stephen Bass and Dean Wengrow and Sarah Oram and Malcolm Dunbar and Phil Howells and Dick Green and Barrett and Kelly and and and it's all –

'*Niven, you fucker!*'

'*Oi-oi!*'

'*We're larging it, mate!*'

'*You wanna split an eight-ball?*'

'*Ten pills. No, twenty.*'

'*Load of old pony.*'

'*They wanted two-firm.*'

'*Fucking dropped them, mate.*'

'*Wants a million for the publishing.*'

'*Here's a fifty, Jocko – pay your mortgage off!*'

Much later, I smuggle some old Irvine pals into the hotel for a few drinks. It's getting very late when the door to the bar swings open once again.

Strummer walks in.

He's playing the following day, with his new band, the recently formed Mescaleros, whose debut album is finally about to come out, 'Techno D-Day' intact. Even a sleeve painting by Damien Hirst will be unable to save it from charting at number seventy-one. (*Ferdy – 'You dodged a fucking bullet there, Niv.'*) We haven't spoken since my telephone sales pitch last year, but, impregnable on lager and cocaine and figuring 'hey, that's showbiz' I call out with a cheery, 'Hi, Joe!'

He comes straight over and joins us, any animosity clearly long forgotten in the whirl and tumble of what it takes to be Joe Strummer year after year. Andy Crone's face almost falls apart, his hand shaking as he reaches for his pint.

We drink round after round and do knuckle bump after knuckle bump of racket. Joe starts openly rolling joints and passing them around. As we get into the early hours, his long-suffering tour manager appears with increasing frequency and tries, gently, to get him to go to bed. No sale. Crone tries to get Strummer onto a diatribe about how terrible festival headliners Blur are, both oblivious to the fact that Blur are sitting maybe ten feet behind them. As dawn approaches, the door flies open once again: Strummer's wife Lucinda is standing there, fists planted on hips.

'JOE! BED! NOW!'

Strummer holds his hands up in surrender and says goodnight. Andy reverently fingers the remnant of the last joint Strummer rolled before heading home.

But there's still a few of the guys in the bar, so it's *'Oi-oi!' 'We're larging it, mate!' 'You wanna split an eight-ball?' 'Ten pills. No, twenty.' 'Load of old pony.' 'They wanted two-firm.' 'Fucking dropped them, mate.' 'Wants a million for the publishing.' 'Here's a fifty, Jocko – pay your mortgage off!'*

No sunlight pierces the basement bar of the Glasgow Malmaison.

'Bye-bye, daddy . . .'

You've noticed it, haven't you? You're a keen reader. You've picked up on a strand emerging throughout this section . . .

Blitzed on cocaine.

Half-hourly trips to the toilet.

Pills and coke and strong German beers and shots.

Fuelled by cocaine and hubris.

And I'd love to be able to tell you that we're about done with this stuff. But we're not. Incredibly, there's a distance left to run.

By 1998, Stephanie had finally moved down from Glasgow and she, two-year-old Robin and I move out of west London and into suburbia, in Berkhamsted, Hertfordshire. Good schools, pretty commuter town. The canal, the high street, the old castle. On weekends it is walks and Waitrose and watching TV. But it is difficult for me to enjoy any of these activities because, on account of my Monday-through-Friday life, I am usually shockingly hungover. And here comes a guy you'd like to drag out of that line-up. I mean, look at him. Almost every night of the week he goes to see a gig. Which involves him in drinking heavily and taking cocaine – often before, during and after the gig – at the newly opened Soho House, or in the Marathon Bar in Camden, or down the Groucho. Later, he crashes out on someone's sofa, or in a hotel room. Or he catches a (very) late train home from Euston. Or, several times, *he drives home.* Having somehow survived the motorway, he will creep in the door in the early hours of the morning, smashed, wired, and stagger into the kitchen, where he guzzles Night Nurse straight from the bottle before tiptoeing past his infant son's bedroom and crawling stupefied into bed next to his wife. He gets up late, hungover and grumpy, and drives back into London where he will do it all over again. *Cheat, sleep, repeat.*

He goes to a show by recent Independiente signing Roddy Frame, at Dingwalls in Camden. And then the dressing room. *('Amazing.*

Amazing. Just gotta use the bathroom . . .') And then the after-party. And then the after-after-party. And then, naturally, the hour-long drive out to Hertfordshire, where, making the long, curving turn that connects the M4 to the M25, he loses control of the BMW 3 Series and hits the barrier on the right-hand side of the fast lane at 70mph. He slews – spinning and screaming – across three lanes before coming to rest on the hard shoulder. Because of the lateness of the hour, there is no other traffic. He sits there, unhurt, but stupefied. He tries to drive away, but the front bumper has been mashed into the driver's side tyre. Sitting on the grass verge in the warm summer night, he calls the RAC and it takes an eternity for the tow truck to arrive. Finally, it does. The tow-truck man asks him no questions and receives no lies. The car is almost fully loaded onto the flatbed when the police cruiser appears, coming down the slip road from the M4, the same way he just travelled . . .

It slows as it approaches them (a sentient beast, snuffling, sensing prey), then pulls over and puts the blinkers on. The breathalyser test is fast and conclusive. The officer's slow whistle through gritted teeth. He is arrested and taken to Hemel Hempstead Police Station, where he spends the few hours before dawn coked-up and sleepless. (It is a minor miracle he does not have the drug on him at this point.) His wife comes to collect him in the morning, their two-year-old son holding her hand, smiling up at him, impressed no doubt by this unexpected adventure, by all the excitement and the uniforms. The sight of his son's innocent face, the thought of what he could have done the night before to someone else's son or daughter . . .

At this point in a certain kind of biography, we usually come to the epiphany, the turning point. The place where the prose tends

251

towards stuff like *'I saw now that I was destroying myself and everyone I loved.'* Towards: *'What had I become?'* It is the bottom rung from which redemption can begin. For a full year after Richard Dreyfuss crashed his Mercedes into a palm tree in Beverly Hills, bent on coke and vodka, the actor said that everywhere he went he was accompanied by a vision of a little girl in a pink dress and horn-rimmed glasses. 'I knew that little girl was either the little girl that I didn't kill that night, or she was the daughter I hadn't had yet. I knew that as a certain fact.'

No little girl, in whatever kind of dress or eyewear, appeared unto this guy just yet. There was no turning point. No. In fact, this maniac goes the other way. He doubles down. Soon after the crash he decides to leave his wife and son, move back to London, and really knuckle down to the business of going completely crackers. No little girl, then. But he still sees the little boy all the time: as a toddler, sleeping as he looks in on him in the early hours, the whisky-cocaine glaze on his eyes, greasy and cracked, like the tiling on the wall of a pub toilet. He still sees the boy tugging on his sleeve to play as he lies wallowing in another pouch-eyed hangover, as he slept away so many mornings of his infancy. I still see Robin (and, yes, enough, let's lose the pathetic armour of the third person) as I left the house in Berkhamsted for the last time, the starfish made by his tiny fingers splayed against the glass of the living-room window.

'Bye-bye, daddy. Bye-bye . . .'

The business of having more children when you are older – when you no longer live the way you did when you had the first children – is salutary. It is dictionary-definition salutary: *'containing, or bringing, a warning'*. An hour spent with my baby son today can bring a jolt as hard and sharp as a box cutter punched into my ribs, as it evokes the hours I didn't spend with my son back then. And Stephanie's voice, as I headed for the car with the last of my bags, saying, *'Please, please don't leave us.'* Still hear it. All the time.

I still leave of course, back in 1998.

And I often wonder how all of this went with Gary over the years. The pain of the absentee father. If you have children who you do not live with, it becomes a part of you. It's not there in every thought, every moment. You can go about your business – you can go see the movie, eat the dinner, drink the drinks – but it's a bit like, when lying in bed at night, I sometimes feel a pocket some-where at the bottom of my lungs that never gets properly filled, no matter how deeply I breathe. The presence of other small chil-dren is an obvious precursor to you suddenly becoming conscious of this space within you, but there are others: the sight, as you buy your newspaper or your cigarettes, of a sweet they liked. The frag-ment of their beloved cartoon glimpsed as you channel-hop. The box in the corner of the restaurant menu saying 'FOR KIDS'. I don't know how all of that went for Gary, but I know how it went for me sometimes, when the sensations of loss, longing and guilt moved from being a background hum to a crashing symphony. Boy, do you look to drown that racket out, as you reach for the bottle, for the wrap, for whatever . . .

When I finally leave London in 2003 and move to Buckinghamshire to try and write a novel, I am within half an hour of Stephanie and Robin and I attempt to make amends, to get closer to my son, who is now seven. And I think we get there in the end, Robin and me. I don't think I was completely defined for my son by my absence. But there are the guys who *never* get there. Who never even try to get there. The guys who sit in the corner of the basement bar that sunlight does not pierce for ten or twenty years, shouting with their friends, braying with laughter, 'staunchly' ordering another round, doing another 'cheeky' bump. And then their red eyes lift from the glass-strewn tabletop to see the waiter approaching, his shirtsleeves wet, his face misted with sweat. Because it's been a long old session, hasn't it? They're closing up now. And in the waiter's hand is a small silver tray. Pressed to it with his thumb, dangling long like an unfurled piece of ticker tape, with its tumbling zeros and obligatory service charge –

The bill. *Ooof.*

Steep.

Yes, ruinous steep was the tab handed to Shades.

PART FIVE

Friday, 3 September 2010

We are gathered again in the family room of the ICU (the dust-furred plastic flowers, the pastel prints, the magazines: a royal in a jungle setting, a breakfast TV presenter's anthracite kitchen) as the doctor explains what will happen this morning.

They are going to extubate Gary by removing the ventilator that has been filling his lungs for him for the last four days. He will then be breathing on his own. It is uncertain how long he will be able to do this for. It could be hours, minutes, days or months. Or perhaps 'indefinitely'. (Linda and I exchange side-eye at this, the worst conceivable outcome.) The doctor suggests we go and get some coffee while they perform the process and they will come and find us when they are finished. The three remaining members of the Niven family head for the cafeteria. The fine weather continues and the hospital, with its acres of glass, its heated wards, is stultifying, tropical. We have just reached the counter and are ordering (Linda and I with our foamy cappuccinos, mum's spartan cup of black filter coffee) when a nurse from the ICU comes running in and up to us.

'I'm sorry, you'd better come back right away . . .'

★   ★   ★

'He started crashing the moment we removed the ventilator,' the nurse tells us as we run back along the corridor. Before we re-enter the ICU we are warned that he may be making unpleasant noises as he struggles to breathe. We are warned, but, even so, my first thought as we come back in is – this can't be real. This isn't serious. Because he's making the worst, the loudest, snoring sounds imaginable: an asthmatic sea lion with a megaphone strapped over its mouth and nostrils. There is also the death rattle coming from his chest, like a bonfire crackling, like the pebbles of a beach cricking and shlocking as the tide re-arranges them. It is horrific. Mum starts to cry.

Gary is drowning from 'excessive respiratory secretion', common in extubated coma patients who cannot clear the fluid that quickly builds up in their lungs. There is also something called 'post-extubation stridor', giving rise to the impression – the illusion – that the patient is struggling, fighting for life. Along with the shock of seeing someone who has been utterly silent for four days suddenly making all this noise, there is the shock of seeing his whole face again, unadorned by the mask and pipe. There are indents next to his mouth, livid purple bruising, like the stains from a night fuelled by red wine, at the right-hand corner of the lips, where the ventilator tube has been resting.

And then there are the numbers and lines on the phalanx of monitors at the head of his bed, Ice Breaker blue and Amstrad green, all tending the same way, spiralling downwards like a stock market crash. I stand at the foot of the bed. Linda sits on Gary's left side, head down, crying, shaking. Mum stands on his right and takes his hand. After a few minutes the hellish snoring subsides, becoming an occasional honk or rattle. His heart rate was in the nineties when we came in. It is already in the fifties. Mum strokes his hair and talks to him. Linda and I are losing a brother, but we are both parents now too, and I know as we look at mum – bent over, her tears falling onto her son's face for the last time – that we are both imagining the same thing: watching one of our own children die. The moment is hyper-real. Too raw to be properly comprehended. It feels like a nightmare, like being forced to watch a horror film that cannot be turned off. Malcolm McDowell with the eye clamps in *A Clockwork Orange*. It feels like the very skin has been peeled from our eyeballs as we watch her kiss his hot, feverish face and hold his hand as, for the second time in her life, she has a conversation with someone taking their last breaths. This time, however, the dialogue is entirely one-sided. Mum is crying hard, gasps and high-pitched sounds are escaping her, but she gets it all out in the end.

'You were my beautiful wee boy, Gary.'

'I'll miss you so much. I'll think about you every day.'

And she says, 'I love you,' over and over.

Look after the three of them.

Now the numbers are in the twenties, flashing and beeping, cockpit instruments in a terminal dive. (*'Terrain! Terrain! Pull up! Pull up!'*) Linda takes Gary's other hand and presses her face into it as she cries. I'm watching the scene as part of it, as a son and a brother, but there is also the writer, who is not quite part of it, who knows that, once this is all over, he will go into the little bathroom down the hall, lock the door, take out his notebook, and record all these details, that months or years in the future, he will have need of them. And here they are now, more than a decade later, in the desk drawer in Buckinghamshire, crabbed red ink (where did *that* pen come from?)

in the black Moleskine. All the things that were said, the sounds he made, that mum made. The wine stain of that bruise. I move around Linda and stand beside him, to the left of his head. The cut, bruised knuckles, the noughts-and-crosses boards of scars on the forearms, contact points in his long war against himself. I cradle his warm face: the scar across his nose, from that party when the house got smashed up, the teenage act of lunacy when he was twenty-five. The broken vessels in his cheeks, blood forced up by the hanging. His right eyelid has flickered open a tiny bit and I can see the eyeball trying to flip upward in the socket, the pupil huge and black, fixed, pretty vacant (*do you remember that? Sitting on the stairs all those years ago, where the echo was good? 'Load of pish,' you said. Is that still in there somewhere, even now locked in a basement room somewhere in your memory palace as it all burns down around you?*), as if he is trying to look up into his own brain, into the organ that caused him so many problems: the splintering headaches, the crazy impulses and the bad decisions. I smooth the eyelid back down and lean in to kiss his forehead. *'Do you think I would leave you dying?'* Well, here we are. I put my mouth to my brother's ear and whisper my own regrets –

'I'm sorry, Gary. I should have tried to help you more . . .'

His heart rate sinks to the teens, into single figures. The hellish snoring has stopped. The monitors flatline. Then, incredibly, one of the screens begins to rally, his heart rate, heading *back up again*, into the twenties, the low thirties. I look over to one of the doctors who is hanging back, a respectful distance across the room, my expression asking – is this a miracle? He shakes his head gently, telling me it is normal, it is the body, doing its body thing, fighting to hold onto life. Another short, abrupt snore, shocking in its volume and suddenness.

260

Electrical impulses, final signals. I lay a hand across his heart. *I'm sorry, wee man – I can't get us out of this.* In a voice that is not quite my own, high and breaking, I say my last words to my little brother.

'Come on, Shades. That's enough now. Time to go, wee man.'

With this benediction, Gary Alexander Niven dies.

It is 4pm on a fine September day in 2010.

He is forty-two years old.

2003

Bentshots and Rentboys

But herein lies one of the great joys of crafting a narrative. Because – just like Travolta's smack-addled hitman Vincent Vega in Shades' beloved *Pulp Fiction* – no sooner have we seen the corpse than here he comes, strolling confidently back into the story . . .

'Haw! Bawbag! Whit utter pishflaps is that yer cooking?'

'Gary! Language!'

'Awright, maw?'

Shades strides large into the family barbecue, in my mum's tiny square of garden, behind the house on Livingstone Terrace. The Roman Emperor-style haircut, a pretty blonde girl on one arm, a case of Miller Lite tucked under the other and a blazing Club dangling from his mouth. He comes over to the grill I am manning. 'Prawn kebabs,' I tell him. 'I marinated them in . . .'

As I crap on, describing the marinade, he is looking at me intently, nodding, stroking his chin – 'mmm, mmm, aye, is that right?' – giving a performance that might best be described as 'impression of a man who gives no fucks, making it very clear he gives no fucks by trying to look like he really gives a fuck'.

'And some minced garlic.'

'Is that right?' Gary replies, eyebrows dancing, fingers drumming on his chin, still faux-fascinated, before he takes a heroic drag on his cigarette and flicks his long ash across the grilling shellfish. 'You are seriously *bent*, John.'

Even someone like myself – a writer who has been accused of every stripe of homophobia, misogyny and sexism – cannot help but be impressed with the depth to which Gary strip-mines the word 'bender' and all its derivatives: bentshot . . . bumboy . . . arsebandit . . . homo . . . rentboy . . . gayboy . . . All of these and more would be hurled at you for crimes as varied as watching the news, reading a broadsheet newspaper, using any 'ism', listening to any guitar band other than Oasis, wearing a dress shirt or a jacket and once, incredibly, for talking about my girlfriend. I stare stupefied at the ruined prawns as, behind me, Gary works his hero's way around the gathering, accepting and bestowing high-fives, throwing out many a 'bender' and 'bumboy' as he goes. This was the language of the time and place he'd come of age in and his position in the community: the 80s, Ayrshire, minor gangster. He also knew it both scandalised and delighted me; the former because Shades had long ago cast me in the role of *Guardian*-reading leftie, and the latter because it showed him living up to the very hilt of the cliché I'd assigned to him: a pure ned banter machine, freshly minting anecdotes for me to take on the plane back to London.

But the wheel of fortune is turning by the time Gary strides into that barbecue. He has steady work on a construction job in Amsterdam. The blonde girl on his arm is Leigh, who will soon be his fiancée and will be instrumental in helping him put prison behind him and get his life back on track. Following their engagement Gary proves he is the bigger man when, over a decade on from my snub, he asks me to be his best man. Possible wedding locations are discussed: Spain, maybe the Caribbean. Gary also decides that the traditional act of simply buying an engagement ring is not enough. A bigger statement is needed: he gets Leigh's name tattooed across his back in huge letters. Except, not quite. In a very on-brand move, Shades does not have 'LEIGH' inked forever into his flesh, he goes with 'LIEGH' instead. She surely gasps when she sees the misspelling for the first time, when he dramatically unveils the masterpiece. Then the pause, before Leigh laughs. 'That's not how you spell it, Gary.'

'Eh? Ye sure?'

She is.

'Ach, it's aw wan.'

Spelling, you may be sure, was also for benders.

The wheel of fortune that has raised him to this pinnacle of soon-to-be-married solvency – what will be the happiest time of his adult life – is well on its way to depositing me at the very bottom . . .

Writing #4

I've managed to fail upwards in the music industry for the best part of ten years, but there's no getting around it: I am a *terrible* A&R man. As the 90s sputter out, I've made a couple of signings I'm proud of – Mogwai, the Pernice Brothers – but nothing that has made a significant dent in the charts. Meanwhile, I throw a demo tape by a three-piece from Teignmouth – the town I was in when I heard my dad was dead – into the wastepaper basket and that's the last the world ever hears of Muse. I laughingly dismiss an Oxford band as 'sub-Radiohead drivel', thus ending the career of Coldplay once and for all. And it's not just that I'm bad at the job, as I get into my mid-thirties I'm becoming terrified at what it might mean if I was slightly better at the job. What then? I'm forty in a bad leather jacket, standing at the back of a gig in Camden on a Tuesday night? Wishing I was at home reading a book? The lifestyle is losing its allure as the hangovers start to bite. What you would have shaken off in a morning in your early twenties is starting to take a day or two as your thirties progress. And there's something else, something that hasn't left me alone over the years, that keeps coming back, nagging and nibbling at me – the joy I got from all those failed hours at the typewriter or computer: the terrible short stories, the abandoned detective novel, the abandoned horror novel.

The manuscripts were abandoned, yes, but the feeling I got when I was doing it, that it felt right, that this was where I was meant to be, that won't go away. But the thought of leaving all the stuff I've enjoyed for so long – the company car, the bottomless expense account, the fat salary, the free travel, the huge mobile phone bills someone else pays – is terrifying. Because trying to get published looks to me very much like the process of bands trying to get signed: the dozen or so acts who 'make it' every year out of the millions of demo tapes. So, without quitting my job, I begin to chip away at yet another attempt to write a novel. It is going to be about the excesses and outrages I have witnessed in the music industry of the 90s. My working title is 'Unrecouped' – the term for the money invested in an act that has yet to be earned back. I grandly imagine that it refers to the balance of the main character's soul. I am writing in the third person, trying to tell a kind of *Candide* story: the innocent abroad who comes into the music business full of hope and who gradually becomes corrupted beyond belief.

And, dear God, it stinks. It reeks to high heaven.

I cannot fully describe how bad this novel is: it is so turgid, joyless and sanctimonious that it is painful for me to read sections of it back. It is way, way too 'on the nose' and just dead, dead, dead. And it occurs to me that there are likely factors hindering the composition process. Like the fact that I'm still living in west London, living the same life I have been for the last decade, the kind that involves the weekend starting on a Thursday night and ending in the small hours of Monday morning.

For I quickly find I cannot write even the bad stuff I am writing when I'm hungover. Trying to summon the confidence and vigour you need to dream a world into being when you're broken with self-loathing is beyond me. Seeing as I'm pissed from Thursday till Monday and then hungover from Monday until Wednesday, it soon becomes clear the arithmetic isn't adding up. A one-day working week isn't going to cut it. So, at the end of 2001, almost exactly a decade after Kevin and I went for that drink in Bar Ten, I leave the music industry to try to write the novel properly. Two things provide the final jolt for the decision, both from Stephanie, my now ex-wife who somehow knows better than I do what needs to happen when she gives me: a) nearly thirty grand in cash when she buys me out of our house in Berkhamsted and b) a Christmas present – a hardback copy of Stephen King's *On Writing*.

I am thirty-five. Forty is on the horizon now.

My new girlfriend Helen and I decide to save some money by (temporarily) moving out of London. We give up our rented flats and move into Helen's family home, a seven-bedroom house in Princes Risborough, Buckinghamshire, about thirty miles west of the city.

We share the place with her mother, Sheila, a retired doctor, and her younger brother, Fintan, a junior doctor in nearby Oxford. In my self-delusion I believe that the windfall from the Berkhamsted house will last a year or two, about exactly the time it will take me to write the Great British Novel.

I am, obviously, insane.

—

December 23, 2003. I'm back in Glasgow for the holidays, Christmas shopping in House of Fraser on Buchanan Street on a very meagre budget, when my (now pay-as-you-go) mobile rings – mum.

'Have ye heard yet, son?'

'Heard what?'

'That's Joe Strummer away.'

'Eh? Away where?'

'He's dead, John.'

I sit down heavily on the edge of a display case as it flies through me: *Craig's bedroom. The Magnum. The Spice of Life. The Groucho.* It all feels personal somehow, Strummer's death tied to my own situation: here in womenswear, with maybe thirty pounds to buy Christmas presents for my son, my girlfriend, my ex-wife, my mum, my sister, my brother. This novel that I can't write and that nobody will want to read anyway.

Oh, Joe, I'm sorry. I'm so sorry. What did I know? It's so hard when you put yourself out there and people say, 'no, thanks'.

'They say it was something to do with his heart,' mum says.

I cover my face with my free hand and cry. 'Aww, son,' mum says. 'He was such a good . . .' She reaches for the word, finds the right one: 'a good *hero* to all you boys.'

—

While I am living with my girlfriend's mum, having cashed out what property interests I have in order to try and become a writer, back in Irvine, Shades becomes a homeowner for the first time. In October 2004, he and Leigh buy a two-bedroom, terraced ex-council house up in Bourtreehill. It's one of the houses that went up in the early 80s, out in the fourth ring of the town, where I used to deliver the milk along half-built streets littered with stacks of timber and piles of roofing tiles.

On a rare visit home, Gary and I go for a round of golf. I drop him off after we play and he proudly shows me around his new home, pointing out the hardwood floor in the living room he has laid himself, the big-screen TV. The Xbox. Linda and I have marvelled at Gary getting all of this together. Getting it together enough to become a homeowner, to instruct a solicitor and have a survey done, to obtain the mortgage, life insurance, buildings insurance and so on. And we sense feminine know-how in this development, Leigh's hand in all of it. For there is a certain kind of man for whom running a home – the bills, the organisation – is all too much.

So, with her help, here's Shades, just a few years out of jail and, against all odds, living the good life, with his trainers up on his coffee table in his own home as we sip beers, his big TV on soundlessly, his

271

fiancée pottering about somewhere in the background. And there's mum's palpable relief that, for now, at least one of her sons' lives is running on track. For I've recently had to borrow three hundred quid from her to insure the car outside, the car I can barely afford to run. For I have burned through all the cash now. Helen is working as a trainee solicitor, and her salary is pretty much supporting the two of us. Our 'temporary' stay with her mum has entered its second year. There are weeks where I find myself putting *three quid* of petrol in the ageing Saab. The shame at the counter, the lie that I forgot my wallet. It's just enough fuel to drive the fifteen miles over to Berkhamsted and back, so I can pick Robin up from school.

'Do ye fancy getting a Chinky in, wee boy?' Shades asks, channel-hopping, uncapping a fresh Bud, enjoying my knee-jerk, liberal discomfort with the word.

Feeling the single pound coin I have in my pocket I say, 'Nah. Said I'd go home and eat with mum . . .'

The Nature of the Beast

But, even in the good times, with things going well, there are problems. The nature of the beast. The nature of Gary. There's a party at mum's house for Linda's thirtieth birthday.

It is high summer and, after all the guests have gone, Leigh and Gary and mum and Linda sit up late into the warm night, out the back by the firepit, talking and drinking. Around 2am Gary decides it is time for him and Leigh to go to bed. Leigh says she wants to stay up for a bit – she's having a good time. Gary gets it into his head that this is some sort of betrayal. That they should go to bed as a couple.

'What is this?' Linda says, laughing. '1952?'

Gary gets angrier, insisting she comes upstairs. Leigh refuses. It escalates, as it so often did with Gary, until he's standing there shouting at her in front of mum and Linda, fists balled by his sides, the veins in his arms and neck cording. Linda looks at him – shouting, drunk, furious – and realises that he very badly wants to hit someone. But the only possible candidates are his fiancée, his mother and his sister. Then they hear voices from out in the street, from Livingstone Terrace. Gary throws the gate open and runs out through the front garden towards the sound: five or six wee neds, in their late teens or early twenties, crossing the street, heading home towards Castlepark after a night drinking downtown.

Shades lurches towards them, arms extended, fingers waggling as though tickling two invisible trout, beckoning them towards him in time-honoured 'come into me' fashion.

'HEY!' he shouts. 'WHIT YOUSE SAYING, YA WEE PRICKS?'

Confused at first, the lads soon get with the programme and Shades gets the outcome he's after – a full-on fight in the middle of the street, fists and feet flying as these boys kick the shit out of him while the three women who he – ostensibly – cares for most in the world stand there, screaming and crying. Fight soon over, he staggers back into the garden – nose burst, eye swollen – brushes past them into the house and storms off to bed, Linda's birthday party ruined, ending like so many other nights have, in tears and blood and *why, Gary, why?* 'It was like an act of self-harm,' Linda will tell me, later. 'Like he knew he'd get beaten up and that was what he wanted. He couldn't hurt us, so he just wanted to hurt himself.'

★ ★ ★

What feels like the bottom for me arrives in the spring of 2004, when I begin to rob Helen's brother. One afternoon, at the desk in the spare bedroom out in Princes Risborough where I am toiling on the book, I am floored by all of it, overcome with hopelessness, with the stark facts.

I am penniless, living with my girlfriend's mum.

I have an eight-year-old son who I cannot support.

I've never had a 'real' job in my life.

I have no marketable skill set.

I am regularly sending sample chapters of the novel-in-progress to agents and publishers and the slew of 'not for us' replies are piling up on the doormat. Helen – and Stephanie – have both been incredibly understanding over the last couple of years but, as those tens and twenties fly out of Helen's purse, as we continue to live with her mum, as I continue to contribute nothing towards Robin's upkeep, the hints have been coming thicker and faster that with my English degree, perhaps teacher training might be a good fit. I sit there and start to fantasise about just running away. I go online (the hiss and brrrrp of the dial-up) and look at rental ads for bedsits in strange cities that I have no connection with – Salisbury, Lancaster, Exeter – and wonder how I could borrow or cobble together the money to cover a few months' rent there. Get a menial job. Write in my spare time. Come back when I have all the things I'm dreaming about: a finished novel, an agent, a book contract.

Suddenly I badly want to get very, very drunk. I *need* to get drunk. However, I do not have a penny to my name. There is not a red cent or a single brass razoo in my account. Not a banknote in any of the trousers and suits I go through, the same suits which had accompanied me on endless nights throughout the 90s. Whose pockets had tolerantly allowed themselves to be stuffed full of damp receipts and gram after gram of cocaine. I wander around the empty house and stroll into Fintan's bedroom.

The bowl on the dresser where he puts all his loose change.

And there's a *ton* of it: fifty-pence pieces, pound coins, even some *two-pound coins*. I liberate fifteen quid and rearrange the pile of slush, covering my tracks. Shamefully, horribly, I catch my reflection in the mirror as I creep out of the room.

I walk to the off-licence, buy two bottles of white wine and ten Marlboros and get absolutely *hammered*.

It becomes a weekly thing. And then Helen and I go to the cinema one evening, to see the new Alexander Payne movie *Sideways* on its opening weekend. I don't know much about it beyond the fact that it's billed as a romantic comedy, a fun, beautifully shot romp through wine country in California.

A *fun romp*?

Jesus Christ.

In case you haven't seen it . . .

Paul Giamatti plays Miles, an aspiring writer who is broke, divorced, turning forty and unable to get his novel published. At one point in the film, on a visit to his mother, he sneaks off to her bedroom and helps himself to some money from a secret stash he knows she has. As he does so . . .

He catches his reflection and looks himself square in the eye – a grown man stealing money from his own mother.

I almost have a nervous breakdown right there in the multiplex. I sit there in the dark, face burning with shame, as though everyone in the cinema must know that this scene is aimed directly at me. I can't go on like this. Something drastic needs to happen. And it does: a plan begins to coalesce in my head. Or, more accurately, a plan from a very long time ago recrudesces. I find myself thinking more and more often of my childhood dream, before punk rock and the electric guitar and bands and the music business. Before all that stuff happened, I'd wanted to be a pilot so badly. To be in the RAF like dad. So . . .

On a whim one night – once again, drunk on stolen wine – I find myself nosing around on the RAF website. I click on 'OFFICERS' and read the requirements for enlisting.

Qualifications: University degree or equivalent.

Age limit: the maximum upper age for officers is 39.

I have a university degree. And I have just over a couple of years left until I turn thirty-nine. Here it was, staring me right in the face, the solution to all my problems. A way to provide for my son and shake off my former life of hedonism and my current one of failure: become an officer in the RAF.

I am going to run away and join the military. It will mean abandoning everything and everyone I know, but what the hell. At least I'll be able to send Robin and Steph some money every month. And Helen will surely understand. I am only dragging her down with me. She'll be better off in the long run.

The following morning another visit to Fin's bedroom – now my personal ATM – allows me to scrape together enough money for the train fare into Marylebone and I wander into the RAF recruiting office in Holborn. A friendly captain gives me a clipboard with a questionnaire and an application form. There I sit, ticking boxes and scribbling in personal details. Of course, I know I'm not going to be

276

flying fighter jets now. I'm way too old. But there are other roles. Perhaps administration?

I see myself in uniform, sleeves rolled up in a tent in the desert heat as I efficiently deal with another batch of paperwork. Or maybe a go-getting lieutenant in the military police? I see myself solving some crime on the base, a murder or a disappearance perhaps. Or there's intelligence officer. There I am, in the snowy compound close to the Russian border, analysing charts and graphs in my wintry greatcoat. What about a pipe? Maybe I smoke a pipe now. What about . . .

What the fuck, a voice in my head says, *are you doing?*

I stand up, drop everything, and run out of there.

Wandering down towards Centre Point in a daze in the spring rain, I find myself in the Tottenham pub, on the north side of Oxford Street, at the corner of Tottenham Court Road, opposite the tube station. Alone at the bar among the lunchtime drinkers, I drain a pint of lager, then order another, working my way through the last of Fintan's change. Looking around at the ornate Victorian wood-work, something dawns on me about this pub: it was in here that Joe Strummer found Guy Stevens and asked him to produce *London Calling*. This would have been in the summer of 1979, just a few months before I heard The Clash for the very first time in Craig Russell's bedroom, which led to me buying a guitar, which led me to joining The Wishing Stones and moving to London, then meeting Steph, moving back to Glasgow and working at Bomba. Then London Records. Then Robin being born. Then, eventually, to here, today, twenty-five years later, sitting in an RAF recruiting office.

Half-drunk, looking in the pool of clear, spilt beer on the mahogany, reaching back through the years, I see the reflection of that thirteen-year-old boy staring back at me, sitting lost in wonder on the bedroom carpet of a council house in Castlepark, thinking that this music sounded like the beginning of a great adventure. And I realise that I owe him something, something I have squandered along the way.

My best shot.

Whatever I have been doing so far isn't nearly enough.

I am going to have to work much, much harder.

If every successful novelist has two or three failed, unpublished books stuffed in their desk drawers, then I am just going to have to get those books written and out of the way fast, in months, not years. I do not have years. Well, I have two of them, in the spring of 2004.

'If I don't have a book published,' I tell Helen when I get back, 'before I'm forty, then I swear to God, I will go and become a teacher.'

Nadir

When things get bad, the great philosopher David Berman once noted, they get really, really bad.

One morning in April 2004, I am woken in the early hours of the morning by a headache. It is *agonising*, located directly behind my right eye. It feels like someone has driven a splinter through my eyeball and into my brain. The pain increases, like someone is turning up a dial, and I find myself getting out of bed and going downstairs, where I shuffle around, pressing the heel of my hand into my eye socket and whimpering. My temperature rises until I am lightly sweating. My eye is weeping. I feel sick. Weak. It reaches a crescendo of agony after about forty minutes. It is by some distance the worst pain I have ever experienced, and for a moment I fear I may be having a brain haemorrhage. And then – just as suddenly as it started – it stops. Vanishes completely. I look around, shaking my head, blinking, sweat cooling, unable to quite believe it is gone. I have never suffered from migraines and wonder if this is what that was. But don't they last longer? I think something like, 'Jesus, that was weird', crawl back into bed next to Helen and go back to sleep. Only to be woken again a couple of hours later with the exact same headache, only worse this time, even more intense. Back downstairs again, the pain becomes so severe as to be almost unbearable. 'No, no, no, no, no,' I moan, close to banging my head off the wall. And again, just as suddenly as before, it stops completely. I try to drift off to sleep again – it's now close to dawn – but whenever I do, I can feel the shadow of the headache circling my skull, trying to come back, as though the very act of falling asleep itself is triggering it.

It happens the following night and the night after that: an hour or so of sleep before being woken by an agonising headache that lasts for somewhere between twenty minutes and an hour. Then another attack, waking me in the early hours of the morning, the splintering, stabbing pain behind the right eye strong enough to make you want to split your own skull open. The raised temperature, the weeping eye. I am crunching Nurofen like M&Ms. Handfuls of aspirin. My bedside is littered with ravaged blister strips of paracetamol. All to no avail. Nothing works. On the fourth night, weak and broken for lack of sleep, downstairs at the computer between bouts, I take my symptoms to the Internet, where Google quickly leads me to the following:

Cluster Headache (CH) is a neurological disorder characterised by recurrent severe headaches on one side of the head, typically around the eye. There is often accompanying eye watering, nasal congestion, or swelling. These symptoms typically last 15 minutes to 3 hours. Cluster headaches are named for the occurrence of groups of headache attacks (clusters). CH attacks often awaken individuals from sleep, typically striking at a precise time of day each morning or night. They have been referred to as 'alarm clock headaches' because of the regularity of their recurrence and have also been called 'suicide headaches', with some female sufferers describing it as 'worse than childbirth'.

I sit there, dumbstruck, horrified, sweating now with apprehension and fear. I have never had a bad headache in my life. How can this suddenly be happening? Where has it come from? How long will it go on for? I read on:

The cause is unknown. CH affects about 0.1% of the general population and usually first occurs between 20 and 40 years of age. Men are affected about four times more often than women. In episodic cluster headache, attacks occur once or more daily, often at the same time each day, for a period of several weeks, followed by a completely headache-free period lasting weeks, months, or years. Approximately 10–15% of CH sufferers become chronic, with multiple headaches every day for years without remission . . .

'*Multiple headaches every day for years without remission.*' This is truly terrifying. And, based on my experience of the last few days, possibly something you could not survive. '*Suicide headaches.*'

That morning I go to my GP, who agrees that I am 'very likely' suffering from cluster headaches. He explains that, for this condition, painkillers like the ones I've been taking are the proverbial shooting-an-elephant-with-a-potato-gun. There's a range of treatment for CH, none of them completely successful. At the upper end of the scale, oxygen therapy can alleviate the pain of the attack, but it involves breathing oxygen through a high-concentration mask at a flow rate of two to fifteen litres per minute. Instead, he prescribes a Sumatriptan nasal spray. It turns out that the spray abates the attack while it is happening, but it also seems to increase their frequency. I quickly abandon it altogether and take to suffering through. You watch the clock and begin to get to grips with the fact that, after an hour at most, and usually twenty to thirty minutes in my case, the attacks completely stop by themselves. Over the next two months the headaches increase in their savagery and regularity. I sometimes have five or six episodes a day. I am exhausted, wrung out. Spent. Falling asleep during the day. I go to bed every night full of dread. Sleep becomes your enemy, because you know what it will bring.

And then, the headaches stop.

They vanish just as suddenly as they arrived, and will not return for three years, and never in the severity of this first bout. During the period of the attacks, I've joined an online forum called OUCH: the Organisation for Understanding Cluster Headaches.

The message board on their website is a godsend. It is full of helpful souls who are – or who have been – going through exactly what I have been. And there are some who have it much, much worse: the chronics. The unfortunates whose daily bouts last for months and years on end with little remission. I am staggered by the courage of some of these people.

Another phrase strikes me on the message board.

'Family history.'

Last Orders at the Last Chance Saloon

Christmas is looming. And this year, the end of my third year of full unemployment, it really does feel like a 'looming', the approach of 'something unwanted and unpleasant'. I do not have enough money to buy my son a present. I am girding myself to go begging from friends and family.

The year before, 2003, an editor called David Barker at Continuum Books in New York had launched a new series called 33⅓: short, pocket-sized books that were detailed critical studies of classic albums. He had published six titles that first year, five journalistic deep-dives on records like Love's *Forever Changes* and Neil Young's *Harvest* and a coming-of-age novella soundtracked around The Smiths' second album *Meat Is Murder*. It was brilliant and it happened to have been written by a friend of mine, Joe Pernice, whose band the Pernice Brothers were one of the last signings I made before I left the music industry. Joe put me in touch with David and, back in the summer, I submitted a pitch for a work of fiction like Joe's, but set in Woodstock in 1967, around the time Dylan's backing group The Band were making their first album. This was almost six months ago and I've pretty much forgotten about it when, on a Friday afternoon, an email arrives. The subject header reads: '33⅓ DECISIONS.' I sit there for a long, long time, unable to open it, before I take a deep breath, click, and look at the screen through splayed fingers, eyes half-closed in terror. The wee boy watching *Jaws*. And then the reverse zoom is happening, the background swooshing as the camera gives a seasick, disbelieving lurch towards the words humming on the screen . . .

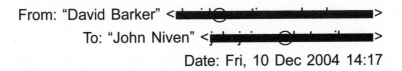

From: "David Barker" <████████████████>
To: "John Niven" <████████████████>
Date: Fri, 10 Dec 2004 14:17

Dear John
I'm very pleased to be able to tell you that your proposal for a book in the series, on "Music from Big Pink", has been approved by the Board here.

I'd like to get your contract drawn up and sent out to you as soon as possible, so please email me back quickly to confirm that you will definitely be able to meet your deadline

of October 1st 2005, and to send me the address to which
we should send your contract.

Very best wishes – and I look forward to working with you
on this book.

David

I sit there, barely able to comprehend good fortune winking at me
for the first time in such a long time. Anyone out there – among you,
the dear, the gentle – trying to write that first book, trying to quiet
that voice saying *no one will care*, may you all get an email like this
once in your lives. I will be writing the book for a micro-advance, a
few thousand dollars, but I don't care. *Something* might happen.

As the wheel of fortune nudges me up for the first time in a long
time, naturally someone else has to clunk down.

'Och, Ah don't know what happened, John, son . . .' Mum is using
her sad, world-weary voice. 'You know Gary. You cannae get much
out of him.'

Just a couple of years after they bought the house together, everything
changes: Gary and Leigh split up and she moves out. I call him and,
like mum, don't get very far. 'Ach, nae big deal, John. Better aff so
Ah am. She was doing ma heid in.'

'But what about the house? Are you going to sell it?'

'Naw! Am Ah fuck. Ma hoose.'

'But doesn't Leigh own half of it?'

'Said she wiznae bothered. Said Ah can have it.'

284

'But, won't she still be on the mortgage? The deeds? She—'

'Naw. Ma hoose,' he repeats firmly.

'Yes, but legally you need to—'

'She's the wan that's left! No me! It's ma hoose!' He starts to get angry, flustered and irritated, as he always does when confronted by anything technical or legal. 'Ah've done aw the work tae it so Ah huv!'

'Gary, listen. If Leigh doesn't want anything to do with the house, that's fine. But legally she still co-owns it if she's on the deeds. You need to go and see a lawyer and fix this. Get the deeds changed.'

'Aye, costs money, but.'

'Look—'

'Aye, aye, awright. Gies peace, John. Ah've got tae go, ma heid's killing me so it is . . .'

He hangs up.

Helen thinks it'll cost a couple of hundred quid to have a Scottish solicitor amend the deeds and that Leigh will have to co-sign, so he'll need to talk to her. I send Gary a cheque for the £200. Leigh had gone, he was there. That was all there was to it as far as Shades was concerned. But, for me and Linda, there was now the fear of how this might all go: Gary, paying his own bills, cooking, cleaning, running his own life. He's been working as a self-employed carpenter and it is only later that we find out how things were starting to go for him at this point. About the job he undertook laying a wooden floor for our Aunt Emily. How he was paid upfront and then the job went unfinished as he disappeared for days on end, claiming 'illness', then reappearing looking 'aff his heid' and suddenly needing more money for 'materials'. How, when the job finally was finished, it was all wrong, badly done, and Shades was nowhere to be found. About the friend-of-a-friend who paid Shades a deposit to fit a kitchen for them and how he then vanished with the money, only finally repaying it after the friend-of-a-friend turned up at Gary's door with a crew threatening violence. About the increasingly angry messages on his mobile phone, messages I will hear after he dies, from a man who'd paid Shades money for a job that was clearly never completed. About arrangements he makes to see mum that are mysteriously broken at the last minute with no explanation. At Gary's funeral our friend Tony Scott will tell me about hiring Gary for a big carpentry job on some flats he was developing, about how Gary would only turn up intermittently and looking 'aff his heid'. Tony will say to me, 'Ah swear tae God, John, Ah was scared tae leave him oan the site some days . . .'

The Central Theme

My debut novella – *Music from Big Pink* – is published at the end of 2005 and is warmly reviewed in *The New York Times*. This doesn't help to sell its follow-up. The next book I am working on is a very different proposition: less sepia-tinged and more blood-splattered. The rejection letters from publishers pile up along with my overdraft statements and credit card bills. Reactions to *Kill Your Friends* range from the commercially cautious (*'we're not sure there's a market for novels about the music industry'*) to the downright horrified (*'this is the most appalling character I have come across in twenty years'*) but my new agent Clare is fuck-them-if-they-can't-take-a-joke ebullient throughout. Even so, as we get towards the end of 2006, it is becoming very clear that we are running out of places to go, and I find myself starting to think more and more regularly about another solution altogether . . .

And we're back to the main subject, the central theme: the last cry from the loneliest place. Most of us have some experience in the realm of suicidal ideation. From the high-school break-up (Fintan once told me he'd lost count of the number of teenagers he'd seen in A&E who'd wrecked their livers during the botched bid with a tub of paracetamol) to the financial meltdown, to the career catastrophe, most of us entertain the stray thought at one time or another. But most of us remain amateurs. Unpublished. Unproduced. As *another* penniless Christmas appears on the horizon, I find myself thinking – daily – about how it might be done. Drowning terrifies me. Jump in front of a train? But the poor driver. Hanging would entrain someone you love having to find the body and take you down. Drugs? I have experience in this realm. Get a load of heroin and – bosh? But I managed to get through smack-drenched London in the 90s without touching the stuff. I'd need someone to show me how to prepare it. Even then, how can you be sure of the dosage? I foresee a scenario where I somehow fail to kill myself but succeed in becoming addicted to heroin. Christmas – borrowing money again to buy a gift for my son.

It is this thought that slams the door in my face. That shows up these thoughts for the self-indulgence that they are. It is tempting to say something glib, something along the lines of 'once you have children, suicide is off the menu'. Tempting, but untrue. Because parents kill themselves every day. William at primary school. His dad did it in the garage with the hosepipe and the engine running. I remember looking at him in the playground and thinking about his dad doing this and wondering how he could keep walking around, how he could keep going, with this knowledge in his head. How did he survive it? All the images I have been toying with – the warm bath and the razors, the sudden leap from the train platform, the walk into the freezing sea, pockets full of stones – cannot survive remembering this. They are supplanted every time by another image: that of Robin's ten-year-old face, broken and bewildered. I see all the birthdays and Christmases I will miss. I see his drinking problem. I see him in therapy. I see the hole in the world next to him, where I should have been. I come up with another scenario that brings some comfort, that helps me get to sleep at night: I'll scrape along for another decade, until he's twenty-one and then he's on his own and maybe I can just drink myself to death. Then – and, once again, incredibly, this happens two weeks before Christmas – the phone rings. It's Clare.

Random House want to publish *Kill Your Friends*.

Family History

It's the evening of Saturday, 1 September 2007, and Linda is with her pal Kirstie, arriving at the Connect Music Festival on the banks of Loch Fyne, where Jarvis Cocker, Mogwai and the Beastie Boys will perform. They've collected their passes, popped back to the hotel to drop their bags, and are just arriving back at the festival site when Linda gets a call from Shades' best pal Stevie. There are nerves and urgency in his voice.

'Linda? Aye, sorry to bother you an that, hen. But, it's Shades. I'm up at his place, and Ah don't ken whit tae dae so Ah don't. He's in an awfy state. Banging his heid aff the waw so he is. He . . . he's talking about . . . Ah don't know. Ah'm feart tae leave him so Ah um. Ah'm worried he might be going tae dae something daft. If ye know whit Ah mean. Ah've got tae go soon and Ah don't want tae lee him alane. Ah didnae want tae call yer maw, ken?'

Linda and Kirstie leave the drizzly festival without seeing a single band, get in Kirstie's car and begin the two-hour drive back down the west coast of Scotland to Irvine. Linda calls me on the way and tells me what's happened.

'He's suicidal?' I ask.

'Stevie thinks so. These migraines he gets . . .'

The alert reader will be way ahead of 2007 me.

That 'ma heid's killing me' that Shades signed off with. Mum's mention of 'Gary's headaches'. I have been so lost in my own drama and failure that I have failed to put the simplest two-and-two together. Thankfully, my financial situation has improved to the point where I can jump on a plane again.

It is the Sunday evening when I collect mum and Linda at Livingstone Terrace and drive up to Gary's house. Linda and Kirstie had got there in the early hours of that morning to find Gary dazed and incoherent. He kept leaving the room and going upstairs, re-appearing more glazed and distant than before. And from upstairs, they'd hear his barks and yelps of pain as he smashed his head against the wall. Gary is embarrassed, angry at first, when he opens the door and sees mum and me there. He looks appalling, unshaven, dishevelled and ragged. He disappears upstairs and we hear the same sounds Linda heard earlier. The house reeks of strong weed.

Mum sits on the sofa, wringing her hands. The house, since Leigh's departure a year or so ago, is neat and tidy enough, but has a spartan, unloved feel. There are just the two pleather sofas facing the big TV. The *Scarface* poster on the wall. No rugs or plants or cushions. The fridge is empty save for a half-bottle of Buckfast chilling in the door. Finally, Gary reappears. It's clear immediately (to me and Linda at least) that he's been upstairs self-medicating with something far, far stronger than weed: the pupils are tiny, pinned, like they were that time in Barlinnie, a decade before. Even so, the smack isn't enough to dull what I know now is happening inside his head. He sits down on the sofa, next to mum, trembling, his temples clutched in his hands, just staring at the floor. I ask him to describe his headaches, the symptoms, how they come on.

'Like, behind ma right eye. I get aw hot. Then it's like a knife intae ma brain. Goes on for aboot an hour then stops. Then comes back when I fa' asleep.'

'Who told you these are migraines, Gary?'

'Doctor.' Pronounced in the full Ayrshire: *'doak-tar'*.

And I picture him in the surgery, in Irvine. His sullen, minimal descriptions of his pain. (*Jist, like, a headache, ken whit Ah mean?*) His submission to authority, to education, as he accepts the overworked GP's knee-jerk analysis of 'migraine'. I find myself thinking of something else I read three years earlier, when I was first going through exactly what Gary is going through now: *'individuals with Cluster Headaches typically experience diagnostic delay of around seven years.'*

Seven. Years.

Because you don't own a computer.

Because you can't use Google.

Because you say things like, *'Aye, jist like, a really bad headache, ken, doctor? Jist really sair.'*

'What have you been prescribed for them?'

'Nurofen.'

'Jesus Christ.'

Like rubbing aloe vera onto third-degree burns.

'How long has it been going on for? This bout?'

'Eh? Months now. Every day. Every few hours.'

'How many pain-free days have you had in the last year?'

'Hardly any. Nane.'

I feel my stomach lurch. It's so appalling I almost want to laugh.

Because it feels incredibly Shades-like. Gary can't just get cluster headaches, can't simply fall into that 0.1% of the population. He must get the most extreme version: chronic cluster. Affecting approximately 10–15% of that 0.1%. These are the damned. Those who will have *'multiple headaches every day for years without remission'*. Who *'hesitate to make plans because of the unpredictability of the pain schedule'*. Who end up with *'anxiety, panic disorders, serious depression'* and *'social withdrawal and isolation'*. Who end up . . .

'You don't have migraines, Gary,' I say, genuine anger rising now. 'Your GP is a fucking idiot. You're suffering from cluster headaches and we're going to sort this out. It's going to get better from now on, I promise.'

Gary looks at me with tired crimson eyes.

The pupils made by the quickest jab of a pencil.

PART SIX

Saturday, 4 September 2010

The italicised, adrenalised aftermath. There are tasks for me and Linda to perform: the death to be registered, friends and family to be called, insurance and property documents to be gathered, bank accounts to be closed, the funeral to be organised. For mum, there are forty-two years of memories to be audited, to be filed and sorted, the worst ones banished, the best to be polished up, like bright stones plucked from a rushing stream.

We take a case of wine up to the hospital, as a gift for the staff who looked after Gary in the ICU. For them, we have nothing but thanks and admiration. With those further up the chain, things are becoming more complicated. From simple denial to outright obstruction, there has been a sense of ranks closing, especially when we learn that another patient in the hospital had killed herself on the same day as Gary: another psychiatric admission who had also been placed unobserved in a room chock-full of ligature points. I make a Freedom of Information request for the transcript of Gary's 999 call. And am turned down. I apply again. A thought has begun to haunt me that I will learn is archetypal when it comes to suicide – if he could somehow have got through that terrible night and into the dawn, would he eventually have turned a corner and found a way forward? Or was the course he was on set, inexorable? And always – *what went on that night?*

Linda and I return to Gary's house to look for some documents we need, and to look for fresh clothes, the clothes he will wear in his coffin. I'm standing in the hall when there's a knock on the frame of the open door and I turn to see a man, maybe in his late fifties, standing there.

'You're Gary's big brother, eh?'

'Yeah, John,' I say, shaking hands.

He introduces himself as a neighbour and says how sorry he is to have heard Gary has died. (It's a small town and the jungle drums have been fierce.) As we make small talk, he reveals that I was in the year above him at school, that he is closer to Gary's age than mine, in his early forties. The sallow yellow skin, the nuts and raisins of his teeth, the slurred, medicated-sounding speech telling a similar story to the brown, stained pebbledash around us that was once glistening white: that the living has become harder around here. Linda comes out of the garage, where she has been having a last look around, and the neighbour nods towards the open garage door. 'Aye, Ah saw him in there wan Sunday, no that long ago,' he says. 'He was in there daeing some work on something, so he wiz. Hud aw his tools oot. He had his wee ghetto blaster oan, belting oot the old Pink Floyd, "Comfortably Numb", ye ken?' Like many of his friends, post-rave, as they got deeper into the weed, Gary had become a big fan of the Floyd.

'He says to me, "See this song? This'll be playing at ma funeral, so it will." Ah said to him, "Fuck sake, Gary! Bit morbid, wee man!" Aye . . .' He looks sadly into the empty garage.

Talking about his funeral to a neighbour just weeks earlier? *Hud aw his tools oot.* It dawns on me that there are no tools in the garage. Or in the house. In the kitchen, stuffed in a drawer, we find a sheaf of crumpled paperwork.

The pawn ticket for his tools.

It is from the Cash Generator shop in the Bridgegate, just at the entrance to the mall, to dad's mall, and it's dated 23 August 2010: eight days before he hanged himself. He pawned a power sander, a power drill and a couple of saws for a total of £45. The agreement gave him the right to buy back the tools up until 20 September for £58.50. Like his purple electricity key, it is the kind of high street usury practised upon the very poorest. There's another pawn ticket, for £150, from the gold shop at the Cross, for the thin chain he wore around his neck, also dated 23 August.

Then, below all of this, we find the deeds to the house. The first thing I notice, on the title page, is that the property is still jointly owned by Gary and Leigh. Whether he couldn't be bothered organising it, or whether he simply wanted to keep the two hundred quid I sent him, Gary had never got around to having the property transferred into his own name.

I can easily imagine him thinking – in his nighttime musings, his pre-dawn flirting with the stepladder and the noose – that mum, who he had fallen into such debt with, would at least benefit financially from his death. That she'd get the house. As he has died intestate, his estate, such as it is, will go to Nina, to be held in trust until his next of kin, Dale, now thirteen, turns eighteen. And this is right and just, as Gary had hardly contributed a penny to the boy's upkeep for the last thirteen years. But I doubt very much, looking at the deeds, that the house will now form part of the estate, seeing as a legal co-owner of the property is still very much alive. This theory is confirmed a few hours later, at the bank, when I show the documents to the girl closing his accounts down.

'Who's Leigh?' she asks, frowning at the deeds.

'His ex-fiancée.'

'Well,' she says, rapping the papers smartly on her desk, 'she's just won a watch, hasn't she?'

Out on the high street, Linda says, 'Can you imagine his reaction?' Unable to help ourselves, we fall about laughing, both of us picturing Gary's spirit, freshly departed, learning that everything he has in the world will be going to two of his ex-girlfriends, picturing the sunderings and smashing-ups going on as the garage walls of the afterlife are punched into splinters.

One further lowering task awaits me. We get a letter from Strathclyde Police informing us that Gary's personal effects – the things he had about him at the time of his death – are ready for collection from Kilmarnock Police Station. I make the fifteen-minute drive eastwards across Ayrshire and park in front of the station. I sign the form at the desk and I sit down and wait. A few moments pass before the sergeant reappears. He places a large, heavy-duty, clear plastic bag on the counter. It would comfortably contain a medium-sized dog. Stamped in dark blue type on the clear plastic are the words 'Strathclyde Police – Evidence'.

I thank him and take the bag out to the car, where I find a parking ticket gleefully tucked beneath the wiper. Using the car keys, I slice the bag open. Immediately I'm hit by a stale, packaged version of

Gary's smell – aftershave, the upper end of department store colognes: Jean Paul Gaultier, Armani or something. It would have been a brand name. Like the clothes I am now taking out. His Armani jeans. His Stone Island parka. His black Adidas trainers. Small. Size seven. And now, most terribly, I am taking out his grey skinny-ribbed Ralph Lauren sweater.

The instrument of his death.

It is still roughly knotted in the configuration that killed him: the arms forming their makeshift noose. The front and side of the sweater, the part that would have been under his chin, is covered in saliva that has dried and crusted into a milky-white residue. I clasp my hands and look out of the windscreen at Kilmarnock as I try to control my jaw, as I let my thoughts do what they will, picture what they will. But even the sweater is not the most terrible thing here. There is one more item, a hell-within-a-hell. Deep inside the large evidence bag is a smaller one. The same clear plastic, the same blue lettering. This one contains the things he had in his pockets when he died. I take them out and set them on the passenger seat one by one, hearing the voice of Frank Oz's policeman giving Louis Winthorpe his possessions back in *Trading Places*.

One disposable plastic lighter. Orange.

One metal tobacco tin.

One set of house keys.

One Nokia mobile phone. Battery dead.

Three pounds and forty-two pence in loose change.

The Frank Oz voice stops. Here it was, all the available cash he had – for we have found none in the house nor any of his bank accounts – £3.42. Gary's net worth at the time of his death. At the

299

age of forty-two. I look at the parking ticket and realise that, as with many interactions with Shades, I am down on the deal. By £26.58. I nearly laugh. But I don't.

I press my head against the steering wheel and cry.

The funeral the following week is packed, as it is for those who go young. There are friends from every walk of Gary's life: school, his various jobs, his adventures in clubland. And some others I do not know, scowling figures in leather jackets, ill-fitting suits and Oakley shades, who keep their distance. Figures from the side of Gary's life we knew less about.

And then, appearing through the crush at the back of the room, looking lost, awkward and bewildered, dwarfed by the horror and enormity of the occasion, by the too-big suit, just like I pictured Wullie Grierson must have looked all those years ago at his father's funeral: Dale, Gary's son, the nephew I meet for the first time that day, born in 1997, when Gary was in prison.

Despite only having been with Gary for a short time, and having been very young when she had him, Nina has done a wonderful job of raising Dale. He is a delightful boy, polite, friendly and bright. It is uncanny the way he so exactly resembles my brother, how precisely he fills the space left by his father, the way the DNA flickers through him, especially around the eyes, because Dale is thirteen and his eyes do what those of any teenager in exclusively adult situations do – they dart, nervous, awkward, finding it difficult to hold your gaze. Months later, I will take him to Ireland for a few days with my son Robin, the cousin he has never met, who is just eighteen months older than him. On the golf course in Kilkee, you see Gary's swing encoded in his son's. And more than that – the ghost of the electrician too.

Afterwards, for the reception, we have hired a suite at the Gailes Hotel, out by the Glasgow and Western Gailes golf courses. It is another fine day, the record-breaking September continuing, and everyone is out on the balcony, drinking, smoking and reminiscing. There's Drew and Bell and Emily and David and Kevin and Amanda and Basil and Graham and Keith and Gordon and Peter and Basil and Tony and all the Andys. And in the middle of it all, as night starts to fall: mum. With her faraway look, her hands lying limp in her lap as she twists the gold wedding band that had been placed on her finger by dad in Fullarton Parish Church, just five minutes away, along the main road, in the summer of 1965, her eyes wide with possibility as he lifted her veil, her twenty-two-year-old heart bursting, racing, eager to run after all that lay ahead of them. Five minutes in the opposite direction from the church: the crematorium, where husband and son were both turned into skeins of ash that drifted into the sky over the Firth of Clyde.

Dad at the end of April.

Gary at the beginning of September.

Their deaths now forever bookending our summers.

Two weeks later, I am back home, at my desk down in the garden office on a Monday morning, trying to settle back into a routine, trying to resume work on the book I am close to finishing, my fourth novel in five years, when my phone rings. Linda.

'Fuck him, the piece of shit. I'm glad he's dead.'

'Wait, slow down. What's happened?'

For the last few years, mum has kept a ceramic piggy bank in the living room. It is the old-school kind that has no rubber stopper in the belly: you must smash it with a hammer when you finally want to get the cash out. It was a birthday present from Gary, and mum had been stuffing it with the money she earned from the massage sessions she'd been giving in the last few years, after she completed her aromatherapy course. Ten pounds here, twenty pounds there, the notes all stuffed into the wee piggy, the idea being that the money would eventually go towards her retirement from working at the gym. The piggy bank came with a slip of paper you put inside it, where you wrote your name – 'JANETTE NIVEN' – and then the words 'I AM SAVING FOR . . .' where you filled in your goal. For some reason or other, earlier this morning, mum went to move the piggy and noticed that it felt lighter than usual. Puzzled, she picked it up and found out that it was, in fact, empty. There had been over four hundred pounds in there, mum reckoned, all her aromatherapy money for the last couple of years. Someone had come in when mum was out of the house and had methodically chiselled all the money out, getting it through the slot with some-thing like a flat-bladed knife. Mostly ten- and twenty-pound notes, mum said.

Depending on the denominations, I uselessly ponder, there would have been something like thirty of them. This was an enterprise that would have required three things: knowledge of what was in there, time, and a key to the house.

Gary. It could only have been Gary.

Linda is torn between fury and heartbreak. Not about the amount of money, of course. About the nature of the offence – stealing the contents of your mum's piggy bank. I ring mum, who has only heartbreak. It turns out that the only thing left in the piggy bank was that little slip of paper. I picture mum's handwriting on the slip – her trembling ad hoc mix of upper and lower case, the dot above even the upper case 'I'.

'Mum, when did you last put some money in there? When did you last notice it was still full?'

'Just before Marymass,' she says, crying.

According to Irvine tradition, the Marymass festival is always the third Saturday after the first Monday in August. This year it had fallen on Saturday, 21 August, the week before Gary killed himself, the week he pawned his tools and his jewelry. So, he'd gone round to mum's when he knew she would be out, used his key to let himself in, and then stolen her savings. I see him, sat there on the living-room carpet, where we used to play fight with dad. Where we used to watch Steed, Purdey and Gambit. Where the Christmas presents would have been piled up. *He's been! Santa's been!'*

I see him as the notes pile up on the carpet beside him. His occasional, stealthy glance towards the front windows, to make sure the coast is still clear. And then he's pulling something through the slot that is not a banknote . . .

'JANETTE NIVEN: FOR MY RETIREMENT.'

This wasn't solely how mum was going to fund her retirement – it was just to have a bit of extra cash, to treat herself – but how was Gary feeling about himself as he took the notes out? Did he catch sight of himself in the mirror above the fireplace as he stood up? Miles in *Sideways*. Me in Fintan's bedroom. And where was he going with this? What was the game plan? Did Shades have some mad plan to repay the money before she noticed? Some cash-making scheme that didn't pan out? Yet another variant on 'The Sure Thing Goes Wrong'? Did he use the money for one last blow-out, already knowing what he was going to do, figuring he'd be dead before the reckoning came? Or was it to pay off a debt that was not among that manila drift on his dining table? One that was being chased by someone whose collection methods didn't involve red letters? Shades must have known he was the only person who would be fingered for the crime. Did he plan to just bare-facedly deny it? To just try and gaslight mum into submission? Or was he going to confess and beg for clemency? Throw himself on the mercy of the court? *'Maw, maw, don't worry, Ah'll get it back. Ah just needed it fur a couple o' weeks. Ah didnae want tae ask ye 'cause Ah knew ye'd only worry.'*

If you're keeping track, that's another fourteen question marks in the paragraph above, piling on top of all the ones I already have. I'm now picturing the questions I have about Gary's final days and hours as a huge queue of people, something like the famed Saatchi-designed 'Labour's Not Working' poster of the late 70s. The questions are lining up in front of a booth, something like a complaints window. But there is no one in the booth to answer them. There never will be.

Suicide's plutonium: the unanswered questions.

With their near-infinite half-life.

You step off the stool, or the ladder, or the chair, you split that atom, and the chain reaction just goes on multiplying, engulfing everything forever. And it is real end-of-the-line stuff, this: stealing from your mother. Like pawning your jewelry. Your tools. How desperate he must have been. How guilty he must have felt. To have had this final deed rattling around in his head along with all the other final thoughts during those final days.

I want mum to stop crying, so I say, 'The thing is, mum, if he'd asked you for that money, if he'd begged you, you'd have given it to him, wouldn't you?'

'Of course.'

'Well, there you are. He just . . . he couldn't ask. He was too ashamed.'

After I hang up the phone, I send mum a cheque for the stolen money. She refuses to cash it. But I am doing stuff. Fixing things up. *Can you see me, daddy? How well I fill your shoes.* You write the cheques and you take the phone calls. You polish your dialogue and restructure your scenes. Only now and then am I glancing over my shoulder, at the blackness, waiting to gobble me up the minute I stop doing all this.

There is a coda. A few months after Gary's death, mum gets a letter from the police informing her that, when Gary's house was raided a few days before he died, one of the items taken was a little over four hundred pounds in cash, which was found stuffed inside a sofa cushion. The police inform mum that this money was taken as it was suspected to be the proceeds of a crime. Whatever investigation was going on has now been closed and the money will be returned to Gary's estate.

Of course, it's impossible to say if this was mum's savings or not, but it seems very likely, the amount being so close, the theft having occurred a week before his death.

I try to imagine his pain and despair at the time. You rob your mother and then the police kick your front door in and take it all away anyway. Your last, your only hope. And why was his electricity still cut off? You'd have paid that right away, surely? If the money was intended to cover another, more ominous debt, then why hadn't he paid it right away? Why stuff the money in the sofa for days? Or was this debt much larger and the four hundred only part of his outstanding balance? Did he have a plan to get the rest together? Perhaps by pawning stuff? Or was the stolen money earmarked to fund some new scheme or deal? How did the police know to look for it? Or do they go through sofa cushions as standard when raiding drug dealer's houses? Or maybe . . .

Ten new question marks right there.

Hello, friends. Welcome. The queue starts over there.

We might be some time.

Around this time, mum, Linda and I sit down in a conference room at North Ayrshire General Hospital with three officials from Ayrshire and Arran Health Board. We're here to discuss exactly how a suicidal patient was allowed to shut himself in a room festooned with ligature points and hang themselves. The meeting does not start well.

'So, Gary rang 999 because of his cluster headaches,' one of them begins. 'He–'

'Excuse me?' I interrupt.

'Yes?'

'That's not why he rang the ambulance.'

'Err' – they look at one another – 'no, Mr Niven. That's why he called 999.'

I sigh as I reach into the file that I've brought with me and slide a piece of paper across the table. One of them picks it up and the other two lean in from each side to read it at the same time. Their faces begin to colour as they read the transcript of Gary's 999 call, the transcript it took me three Freedom of Information requests to obtain, the transcript where he does not once mention his cluster headaches, where he only talks about being scared, scared that he might take his own life.

'I, umm . . .' the stammering begins.

'You see,' I begin, 'I just want to make sure we're all clear. The entire reason my brother came to the hospital that night was because he was afraid he was going to kill himself.'

'How did you get this?' one of them asks me.

'I'm more concerned that you don't have it,' I say. 'Because how can we trust that you're going to give us a satisfactory explanation of what happened that night when you can't even begin with the basic facts?'

'Umm, we'll have to . . . review our information.'

And I finally think, *I am going to fucking sue you.*

Because months of closing ranks and protecting flanks have angered me. Because of the other suicidal patient who took their life in the hospital on the *same day* as Gary, in very similar circumstances. Because the health board are hiding behind some vague 'systemic failure' apology.

Because – and it takes me a while to understand this – in the wake of suicide, you want to *do something.* All that energy and rage. Lashing out as you swing wildly at all those unanswered questions, surrounding you like demons. Had Gary just climbed that metal

stepladder in his garage, who would you sue? The manufacturers of
blue nylon clotheslines?

But he tried.

Tried to stop himself.

He came to you for help.

2008

Run, Don't Walk

The National Hospital for Neurology and Neurosurgery lies on the eastern side of Queen's Square, in Bloomsbury. Like many Victorian buildings of its kind, the interior now bears little relationship to the handsome sandstone facade. Inside it's a labyrinth of sub-divided rooms, with strip lighting blaring down on the forestry of signage: *Admissions, Outpatients, Surgery, Pharmacy*.

'Things will get better, Gary, I promise.'

Thankfully it is no longer just me making these claims. By the summer of 2008, it is Dr Manjit Matharu, BSc, MBChB, PhD, MRCP, the consultant neurologist at Queen's Square and one of the UK's leading experts in Cluster Headache. I sit in his consulting room with mum and Gary, having picked them up at Luton Airport a few hours earlier. Dr Matharu is about my age, early forties, with slightly greying hair and glasses. He carries the easy manner of the capable professional, and you quickly sense how thoroughly familiar he is with this rare, dreadful condition. It is reassuring just to hear him asking the right questions, nodding understandingly, his pen making quick ticks and notes, as Gary describes the onslaught and

311

frequency of his attacks, the side of his head on which they most often occur, the nature and severity of his pain. All the things his GP never asked him.

I found out about Queen's Square through the OUCH message board, after I told some other regular posters that my brother's cluster headaches had now become chronic and that I feared for his life, his sanity. Run, don't walk, to see Dr Matharu was the consensus. He's intrigued by the fact that Gary and I have both been sufferers, research into siblings affected by the condition being still in its infancy. He prescribes new medications – we will try a variety over the coming months – as well as oxygen therapy, to be used during an attack, to abate it. The oxygen must be breathed through a non-rebreathing mask at a specific flow rate and the cylinders must be refilled at the pharmacy in Irvine. Gary is to keep a headache diary, recording precisely the times, duration and severity of his attacks. Gary shifts uncomfortably at the thought of all this work.

'I'll help you, son,' mum says.

Dr Matharu explains that Gary will have to come down to London regularly for further examinations, depending on how his headaches respond to the different treatments. It is a long journey – Irvine to Glasgow Airport, Glasgow to Stanstead, Heathrow or Luton, and then the drive into London – and one that will be made all the worse when Gary is suffering from a headache, which is almost all the time now. But he bravely agrees to take it on.

Gary has not worked in some time now, so the cost of these trips will be shared by me and mum. (And what awaits you, I wonder, if you suffer from chronic cluster headaches in Scotland, in Wales, in the

312

northeast of England and you do not have the funds for regular trips to London?) The three of us come out into the London sunshine and mum hugs him. 'It's going to be OK, son.'

'Come on,' I say to them. 'I'll take you for lunch.'

Rolling Downhill

About that airy invitation to lunch . . .

Six months earlier, in February 2008, Heinemann finally published *Kill Your Friends*. The reviews have been the stuff of some of the wilder two-bottles-of-wine fantasies I have entertained. 'The best British novel since *Trainspotting*' and on down from there. I'm able to fly back to Scotland more regularly again, and Gary and I start spending more time together than we have in years: when I'm back in Irvine, when I pick him up at Heathrow or Luton and drive him into London for his headache appointments.

On my part, some of this is driven by guilt over the fact that I had been so self-involved I hadn't put two and two together sooner about the kind of headaches Gary was having, all those years he suffered needlessly between my first bout in the spring of 2004 and Linda's phone call in September 2007. By the end of 2008 his condition is improving, and I decide to take my involvement further and fully get Gary's life back on track . . .

'What do you really want to do?' I ask him.

We're in the Yo! Sushi just off Tottenham Court Road, mid-afternoon, with some time to kill before we head over to Queen's Square, just round the corner.

'Eh?' he says.

'With your life,' I go on. 'I mean, in a perfect world what do you see yourself doing with the rest of your life?'

Gary eyes the conveyor belt suspiciously as he thinks about the question, slivers of fish trundling past on their blocks of rice, the pink and red slashes of salmon and tuna, the translucent eel. We're only in here as it's the closest place to the hospital bar Burger King, which I vetoed. Gary is what the folks back home call a 'plain eater'. Sashimi is as likely to cross his lips as a penis or a Hail Mary. He orders katsu. 'Christ, John, Ah don't know. Maybe . . . like a foreman, a supervisor on a building site?'

'OK . . .'

Because now that we're dealing with the physical ailments, it's time to deal with the metaphysical malaise. Gary's problem, by my reckoning, is that he's got no vision of where the second act of his life can go. Having just completed what feels like a successful second act reinvention myself, I'm thinking about what I can do to help him with his.

'Well, it's not astronaut or professional golfer,' I say, in my arrogance. 'This must be doable. What would you need in terms of qualifications?'

'Eh?' Forking his chicken. 'Ah dunno, John. Like HNDs and stuff like that?'

'You'd probably have to go to night school and get some GCSEs first.' The route Basil and Keith had both gone down in their twenties, having written school off the first time around.

'Aye, mibbe.' He looks around at the Londoners with their raw fish.

'But they might take your work experience into account . . .'

I crap on about how we might get him on the path to success in the building industry. Because this is what you do, isn't it? You've

314

been to university, so you think something like, 'Right! Let's jolly well fix this!' You do your research, you get a plan of action together and you buckle down and do some hard work and the universe will respond. Gary sips his Coke and half listens. All the things I don't understand . . .

I don't understand the degree to which he is still helping his prescription medication along in all sorts of ways, with Valium and jellies and powerful hydroponic weed and heroin. (Linda: 'He was nodding out at the table on Mother's Day.')

I don't understand that when he does get the occasional carpentry job, he's increasingly incapable of performing it. I don't understand that what Gary really wants is just to be left alone. If someone could take care of everything and let him lie on the sofa coping with his headaches as best as he can, watching action films and playing on his Xbox and smoking weed and occasionally doing some hardman gangster stuff just to keep his hand in, then that would be ideal. I don't yet understand that some people are incapable of running a life. That the daily treadmill of gas and electricity and water and council tax and life insurance and buildings and contents insurance and mortgage and food and HMRC and putting the bins out and overdraft limits and minimum payments is just way, way too much for some people to handle. That they cannot 'jolly well' get on with anything. I do not know enough about suicide and depression yet. (I'll know a lot more later, when the information is of no use to me.) I do not know – sat there chop-sticking sashimi like an insufferable prick – that the instrument panel has red lights flashing across the board . . .

Male.

Single.

Unemployed.

Living alone.

Early forties.

Health problems.

Financial problems.

Substance abuse problems.

I have not yet seen the Samaritans' Men on the Ropes campaign, which focuses on reaching those most likely to take their own lives, men *over the age of 25, who are unemployed or in manual jobs and who have experienced difficult times such as financial worries or breakdowns in their relationships'*. Men like the one sitting across from me in the sunlit restaurant. I have not yet begun to contemplate the onslaught of depression that will engulf a generation of ravers like Shades as they get older. The vast reserves of serotonin that must have been depleted in the decade from the late 80s to the late 90s, from the first pills to the last jellies, all torched on the pyre of *'whatever you do, just make sure what you're doing makes you happy'*.

I am Captain Edward Smith, standing on the bridge of the *Titanic* on the moonlit evening of 15 April 1912. Sipping lemon tea and looking at the glassy, calm Atlantic.

Everything I know is wrong.

'Or, maybe,' Shades says, coming back into the career conversation, 'I could have ma ain joinery business. Need tae pass ma test first, but. I've done the theory part. Just got tae save up for some mair driving lessons.'

I know he's been keen to pass his driving test for a while now (dad's credit-card-thin patience and Gary's belligerence were a ther-

316

monuclear combination when it came to learning to drive) and decide the time is right to tell him about a surprise I've been saving.

'If you pass your test,' I say, 'you can have my car.'

He looks at me. 'What car?'

'The one I picked you up at the airport in today, you clown. The Saab.' My ten-year-old Saab 900 is a relic from the days of A&R, when it was briefly the chicest thing to have in the late 90s. Following the success of *Kill Your Friends*, I'm planning an upgrade and I don't really need whatever I'd get for the trade-in, so giving it to Gary seems like the right thing to do. 'You can have it. It's yours when you pass your test.'

Silence. Not the effusive thanks I'd been hoping for.

Then I realise that he has tears in his eyes.

'You're gaunnae gie me a *motor*?'

'Hey, it's OK. It's fine. Come on now. I'll drive it up soon and leave it in Irvine. But,' I add, 'you absolutely cannot drive it until you pass your test and we get you insured, OK?'

'Aye, course. Jesus, John. Thanks, pal, thanks so much.' There's a pause. The clatter of the restaurant. 'But . . . it'd be awright for one of my pals to drive it, aye? As long as they've goat a licence?'

Uh-oh. 'A hundred per cent no. It'll be SORN'd until you pass your test.'

'SORN'd?'

'Statutory Off-Road Notification. It means it'd be illegal to take the car on a public highway. It even needs to be parked off-road.'

'Aye, but–'

'Gary, it's a deal breaker. No one drives the car but you, and only after you've passed your test.'

I can see he wants to argue but he says, 'Aye, OK. Thanks, John. I mean it – thanks.'

Later, we're in the Saab, driving back to Luton for Gary's evening flight home. Dr Matharu was pleased with his progress. The oxygen is helping to abate the attacks when he has them and the other medication is beginning to reduce their frequency. Gary is looking around the car, soon to be his. 'When dae ye think you'll bring the motor up?'

'Few weeks. I'll leave it in the driveway at mum's until you pass your test.'

'Ye can jist leave it at ma hoose.'

'It needs to be off the road.'

'Aye, in ma garage, but.'

'I thought you worked in there?'

'No that much. It'll be fine.'

'What's wrong with the driveway at mum's?'

'Och, see the bams you get walking by that hoose these days, John? It'll no be safe.'

'It'll be fine.'

'You've nae idea whit it's like in Irvine now. Ah'm telling ye . . .' He goes on and on, fairly working himself into a lather about vandals, gangs, wee neds. I sense something beneath this, some ulterior motive in his intensity. It's not as if the car is a keying magnet, a brand-new Bentley. But finally, bored of it, I give in.

'OK. It can stay in your garage, but listen to me – it will be *illegal* to take the car on the road while it's been SORN'd. Do you understand? No one can drive it.'

'Aye. Course. Promise. Ah swear.'

We're at some traffic lights, near the airport. As I pull away Gary drains the Coke he's been drinking, puts the window down, and tosses the empty can out. I pull over on the verge.

'What the fuck are you doing?'

'Eh?'

'Go and pick that up.'

'Come tae fuck!'

'I'm not kidding. What the fuck are you doing littering out the car?'

'Fuck sake, John,' he laughs. 'I thought you were a punk.'

'Eh? What are you talking about?'

'You used to be a punk rocker, man!'

'GO AND PICK UP THE FUCKING CAN, GARY!'

'FOR FUCK SAKE!' he screams, kicking the door open and storming angrily out of the car. He returns with the can, furious. 'Whit the fuck am Ah meant tae do wi' it now?'

'Keep it until we get to the airport and then put it in a rubbish bin like a normal person. What's wrong with you?' He mutters some more nonsense about punk rock.

From tearful gratitude to the edge of violence in the space of perhaps ninety seconds. The Shades way.

The Red Mist

The following month, I drive the Saab up and spend a few days in Irvine. Graham Fagen, Gary and I go and play golf.

Now, a round with Gary is always fraught with some tension. Like dad, I am a short-fuse artist. No stranger to the hurled club, the agonised string of cursing, the booted golf bag. But with Gary . . . he has some talent as a golfer, but a tendency to swing much, much too fast, especially when the red mist begins to descend. Today, his round starts well but deteriorates as we go on. He is smoking a powerful joint as he plays, which I feel can't be helping. I make the mistake of offering a couple of tips, which are greeted neutrally at first, then with increasing hostility. Things reach a climax at the eleventh, where the wheels seriously come off the wagon for Gary. He pulls his approach shot left, into thick gorse, and takes a couple of swings to hack it out. Then he thins a chip through the green and stubs the one back, leaving it well short, before turning a two-putt into a three-putt. Graham and I stand there in the awful silence known only to golfers watching someone have a total meltdown. This silence deepens as Gary blasts his *third* putt way past the hole, leaving himself still with a slippery two-footer for something like a ten.

'Just pick it up, Gary,' I finally say, softly.

But he's determined to putt out. Trembling with rage, almost levitating, he lines up the two-footer and pokes it. And leaves it hanging on the lip. A tap-in for a card-wrecking eleven.

'*YA FUCKING HOOR!*'

He screams as he swings his putter at the ball like a polo mallet, aiming to smash it away into oblivion. True to current form, he misses the ball completely, carving a huge chunk out of the green, right next to the hole. In golf, this is atrocious, unspeakable behaviour. Smashing a club into the ground on the fairway or in the rough, even on the tee, is like spitting in football: nasty, frowned upon, but an inevitable part of the game. Tearing up the putting green is more like punching the ref. It's the end of the world. If dad had been here to witness this, I cannot even begin to imagine the severity of his reaction. But dad isn't available, so I do the next best thing – I turn into him.

320

'GARY! THAT'S ENOUGH!' I scream, teeth clenched, jaw set.

His own fury is instant, total: 'SHUT YER FUCKING MOOTH!'

He comes towards me, the putter gripped in his fist, his knuckles white. *Like towards Linda, with that hammer.*

'FIX THAT NOW!' I point to the gash in the turf.

He gets right in my face and jabs me in the chest as he screams, *'YOU'RE NO MA FUCKING DAD, YA PRICK!'* Then he turns and storms off, grabbing his golf bag and pulling it after him like a victim, like a hostage. I look at Graham and sigh. He shakes his head. This had been brewing since the first tee.

It had been brewing for forty years.

No Good Deed

A few weeks later, I'm back home when I get a call from mum, who is in tears, barely able to catch her breath.

'Mum, mum, Jesus – what's wrong?'

'Aw God, son, it's Gary.'

'Christ, what now?'

Mum was out back, hanging washing out, when she heard the wooden side gate open. She popped her head around the corner of the house to see Gary, his key out, about to open the back door. He was surprised to see her, clearly thinking the house was empty. 'Hi, son,' she said. 'What are you doing?'

'Ah, Ah was just . . . gaunnae look for something,' Gary said, immediately flustered, caught. Mum came closer and looked past him, to the front garden and Livingstone Terrace beyond.

There, parked at the kerb – the Saab.

'Gary! John told you! You can't drive that car!'

'Ah wiznae! Ma . . . ma pal was driving! He's just away roon the corner.'

Even mum knew this was bullshit. I'd also told her – and him, many times – that *no one* could drive the car. Gary tried to tell her

322

to calm down, that it was 'aw fine'. Fine that he's driving an untaxed, uninsured, declared off-road vehicle without a licence.

'Gary, John told you no one can drive that car! NO ONE!'

'Ach, gies peace!'

'Give me the keys! You're leaving it here!'

'It's ma fucking car, maw!'

'Not until you pass your test!'

'FUCK SAKE! FUCK IT!'

He *hurls* the keys at mum – who, at this point, is literally paying his mortgage, his flights to London, his *food* sometimes – and storms off, shoving the gate open and marching away, leaving the car abandoned on the street in front of the house.

'I don't know what's wrong wi' that boy,' mum says to me, through her tears.

The declared-off-the-road vehicle is now very much *on* the road. So, I must call Linda, whose husband Brian must drive the thirty miles down from Glasgow so that he can move the car onto the driveway. Gary has now transformed a favour to him into a nightmare for four people. I'm dry-throated with rage as I dial his mobile and get no answer. It's probably a good thing, because when I finally get hold of him a few days later, I'm calmer than I would have been when I am forced to listen to his torrent of utter nonsense about how it wasn't his fault, about how it was an emergency, about how his pal was driving, not him, about how his pal is insured to drive any car because he's on his uncle's policy . . . and on and on and on.

'That's all irrelevant. I told you – it's illegal for the car to be on the road at all.'

'How?'

Wearily, I begin to explain the whole SORN thing again.

'Naw,' Gary says. 'You never said that, John.'

A decade after Gary's death, the experience of watching Donald Trump give a press conference will remind me of arguing with my little brother: the three-second memory span, the imperviousness to logic and truth, the utter shamelessness, the way you end up getting sucked onto their playing field, where you find yourself having to fight to defend the utterly self-evident.

'And where do you get off throwing the keys at *mum*?' I ask. 'Shouting at her? Seriously, what the fuck is wrong with you? Everything she does for you, and this is how you treat her?' (Looking back, writing this now, it is difficult to believe that I was having these conversations with a man who had recently turned forty.)

'Ach, fuck off, ya prick.' Gary hangs up on me.

I give the car to Linda.

Gary never passes his driving test.

Gary Wants What He Wants

In the spring of 2009, after Gary's been seeing him for around nine months, Dr Matharu tells us he wants to do a new series of tests. It's possible they'll take a whole afternoon and into the next morning, so we are advised to stay nearby. Mum's coming down too, so I pay for a hotel in Bloomsbury for the two of them and mum pays for return flights to Glasgow the following evening. In the end the tests are completed on the first day. As soon as we come out onto Queen's Square, Gary immediately begins lobbying, urgently, to fly home that night.

'Listen,' I say. 'Mum's already paid for the flights. They're Ryanair, unchangeable. We'd have to buy new tickets.' The hotel is already paid for too and can't be cancelled at a few hours' notice. Gary goes into a rant about his house, about how he shouldn't leave it overnight if it can be helped. How unsafe it is. Again, I'm told how I don't understand the crime in Irvine. 'Forget it,' I say. 'Come on. We'll go and check you in at the hotel, have dinner and I'll run you to the airport in the morning.'

'Look – Ah need tae get hame!'

'Eh? You knew all along you'd be staying tonight.'

'Aye, but now we don't have to!'

He says this as though I am mad, or simple. Once again, I go through the unchangeable flights. 'If we could cancel the hotel, then fair enough, use that money to cover the new flights. But, to go home tonight, mum's out the original flights and I'd be out for the hotel and the new flights!'

'Please, Gary,' mum says, who has probably been looking forward to a night in a nice hotel in London. 'Let's just–'

'Fuck sake!' he snarls. He thrusts his hands in his pockets and storms off ahead of us, spitting to the side every few yards, as is his way. *Jesus Christ.*

As we wait to check in – in the faded grandeur of the dark wood lobby of one of those old hotels in Bloomsbury – I can see Gary is walking in agitated circles a little way off, texting constantly on his phone. As we're getting the keys from the receptionist he comes over and – incredibly – restarts the campaign to go home tonight. 'Gary,' I say, starting to lose all patience. 'What don't you get here? You're staying here tonight and that's the end of it.'

'I need tae get back tae ma fucken hoose!'

'Why? What's happened?'

'WE DON'T NEED TO GO INTAE THE HOSPITAL TOMORROW, JOHN!'

You could go mad having these discussions.

'Gary, son,' mum says, on the verge of tears now as he raises his voice in the lobby. 'Let's go up to our rooms, have a wee rest, and then–'

The utter absurdity of the situation hits me: Gary, shouting and swearing at the people who are trying to help him. The fact that he would willingly involve both of us in more expense so he can rush back to Irvine to . . . what? To guard a TV and an Xbox?

'Gary, if you can give me one good reason why you suddenly need to get home tonight,' I say, 'then we'll see what we can do.'

'Ma heid's killing me, right?'

'And charging to the airport in the rush hour will help?'

'Please, Gary, just go up to your room and lie down, son,' mum says, scared, desperate now.

'Fuck sake!' Gary barks again.

Finally, I lose my temper. 'Right' – I step close to him, put my hand on his shoulder and walk him a few paces away from mum, growling through the jutting bottom teeth and clenched jaw that belong to our father – 'that's enough. You're staying here tonight, ya ungrateful wee wank. If you want to go home, then fine. But you'll have to find a way to get to the airport by yourself and a way to pay for your flight. OK?'

His eyes: mad, shimmering. The fists clenched by his sides. For a second I think he might hit me. 'Ach, just fuck off.' He shoulders

326

past me, grabs his room key from mum, and storms off towards the lifts. Mum sits down in an armchair in the lobby, rubbing her temples, tears in her eyes.

'Jesus Christ,' I say.

'I'm sorry, son,' mum says. 'I don't know what's wrong with him.'

Gary wants what he wants, I think.

Later, when Linda and I find that secret compartment in his house, I will wonder about that day at the hotel in Bloomsbury. Had something happened? All that frantic texting. Did something suddenly have to be taken care of? Something he obviously couldn't tell us about?

Ah, hello, Questions. Friends. Join the queue.

For the Price of a Stamp

As 2009 goes on, Gary gradually begins to uncouple from the process at Queen's Square. He starts refusing to travel down for his appointments. Mum worries and cries. I apologise to Dr Matharu, knowing how valuable his time is, how many other people there are in desperate need of his help. Only mum sees Gary, when she gets the bus up to his house, to take him some food or some cash. He's trying to manage his medication on his own, but those oxygen tanks are heavy. The routine of getting them refilled is tedious and involves lugging one on a bus from Bourtreehill to Irvine town centre. Increasingly, he doesn't bother. His prescriptions are complicated too and start to go unfilled. Linda and I hear rumours that he's hanging out again with some of the darker characters from his past. But Linda is pregnant and my daughter Lila is just a year old. I now have management in Los Angeles who have sold one of my

327

screenplays and I'm starting to get work rewriting studio scripts. I'm spending more time over there. Linda gives birth to her first child, her daughter Orlaith. I fly up to visit with Lila and Helen, and we bask in the happiness of the clan expanding, of more faces to be spread around the table at family gatherings. However, as the days go by, then the weeks, there is nothing from Gary. Certainly not a gift – no one would really have expected that – but not a visit, not a card, not even a *text*. To a degree, mum runs cover for him. He hasn't been well. His head's been bad. He doesn't have any credit on his phone. Finally, as the weeks become a month, I lose all patience with mum.

'Are you seriously telling me that a forty-one-year-old man can't write a letter? A card? That at no point in the last four weeks has he been able to lay his hands on fifty pence for a *stamp* to congratulate his wee sister on the birth of her daughter? His own niece?' Mum cries. She knows how awful his behaviour really is. I call him but never get any answer. He's gone to ground.

Months later, Linda is down in Irvine, visiting mum with baby Orlaith, when Gary suddenly walks in the front door, having no idea Linda is there. He cries when he sees his tiny niece, full of apologies and regret. And Linda embraces him, letting it go, as you so often had to do in the world of Shades, where standards of behaviour that would be unacceptable from anyone else would somehow have to be accommodated. And, soon enough, early the following year, 2010, Gary needs a favour from Linda. He has some shares in Land Securities, the company dad used to work for, who owned Irvine mall. It's not a lot, just a few hundred pounds' worth, a holdover from dad's will, but he wants – needs – to sell them fast.

Linda says that around this time Gary confessed his greatest fear to her: that he was going to end up 'down Cunny House', slang for Cunningham House, the district council offices where the homeless and the drug-addicted wound up, begging for a roof over their heads.

Obviously, Gary has no idea how you go about selling stocks and shares, so Linda agrees to find a broker in Glasgow and handle the transaction for him. A few days later, she rings to tell him it's all done. He'll get the cheque in a couple of weeks.

A pause. Then an incredulous *'Whit?'*

'You'll get the cheque in—'

'Naw. Fuck that, Linda. Ah need the money now.'

'But, Gary,' Linda says. 'This is how it works. They don't just hand you the cash there and then. They—'

'YA DAFT WEE COW!' Gary explodes. 'AH NEED THAT MONEY NOW! NO IN TWO WEEKS! NOW! YE FUCKEN HEAR ME? NOW! *GET IT NOW!*' Linda hangs up on him and rings me in tears. (And how many, many interactions with Gary now end in tears.)

I call him. In truth, I am very up for this, *desperate* for the confrontation, begging for it. The thought that Linda, who has just returned to work and is dealing with a new baby – the baby whose birth Gary never bothered to acknowledge – has taken the time to help him and has got *this* in return? I'm trembling with rage as I listen to it ringing.

Of course, he doesn't answer.

I try a few more times but, in a now familiar pattern, Gary, having caused outrage, goes off-grid while everyone else reels and hisses with impotent fury. I leave a couple of angry voicemails and then, as it does, life resumes.

The Judge

A few months later, July 2010, and I'm at my desk when the phone rings. Gary. I don't answer. I call Linda first.

'Have you spoken to Shades?'

'No.'

'So he hasn't apologised for screaming at you about these shares?'

'Has he fuck.'

'Right. I'll call you back.'

I step out into the garden, light a cigarette and call him back, cocked and ready. Primed for a fight. This time he answers immediately.

'Right, Gary, listen–'

'Aye, John,' he cuts me off fast. 'Dae ye ken the judge? At the *Sunday Mail*?'

'Eh?' I stumble, utterly wrong-footed.

I had been in Scotland's biggest-selling Sunday newspaper a few times in the last couple of years, around the publication of my novels, and I would soon begin writing a weekly column for it. 'The Judge' was the paper's legal agony aunt, a fictional character who helped readers with consumer-related problems. Gary seems to think the Judge is a real person who I might be personally acquainted with.

'*What?* No.' I say. 'Listen–'

'Can ye get me a number fur them?' Gary ploughs on, cutting me off again. 'See, Ah goat this new telly fae Curry's, but they sent the wrang wan, so they did. And they're claiming that Ah cannae . . .'

I look dumbstruck at the phone in my hand – just like they do in films – as the madman rants on. I'm trying to take in the fact that, after everything that has happened recently – after the car, the new baby carry-on, the shares-selling fiasco – it seems that the reason he is finally getting in touch with me is to try and enlist my help in getting a fictional consumer-advocate figurehead from a tabloid news-paper on board with an Erin Brockovich-style legal crusade against a well-known electrical retailer.

What the fuck?

'Gary,' I finally manage to cut in, 'just let me stop you there. I need to be very clear – call Linda now and apologise for the way you spoke to her about these shares.'

'Eh? Whit? Ah didnae–' he begins his denial.

'Shut up. Listen. In fact, I'll go you one further, I have no interest in speaking to you again until you sort this out. Call Linda, apologise, and, until you have, just fuck off.' I hang up on him. I see his number coming up again, but I switch the phone to silent as I step back inside and throw it on a chair, being in no mood to hear him threatening to cut my throat or whatever. *I have no interest in speaking to you again.* And I wouldn't.

For a glance at the timeline here would tell you that we are now just weeks away from Gary's last night on earth. From me walking into the kitchen and seeing Helen cradling the baby Lila and holding the phone towards me. I sometimes tell myself that the last words I spoke to him were the ones whispered to his body in the ICU, as the life left it – '*I'm sorry, I should have tried to help you more.*' But that's not true.

'*Just fuck off.*'

The real last words I spoke to my brother.

331

TEN YEARS LATER

1 September 2020

The tenth anniversary of Gary's coma and death falls during a respite in the lockdowns. I fly up to Scotland to spend some time with mum during what I know will be a difficult week for her. Driving into Irvine from Glasgow Airport, I must remind myself not to automatically follow the route to the old house at Livingstone Terrace. I come in the glass front door and throw my bag down in the bright, spacious hallway, calling out to mum, who I can hear in the kitchen of the big, detached house. The Graceland of our childhood.

Aunt Bell died in 2013, just a few months after mum's seventieth birthday party, which was to be the last big event with many of the family's old guard: Aunt Emily dies the following year and Uncle Drew the year after that. Our cousins – David, Kevin and Amanda – decided to put the Whyte Avenue house on the market in 2018. I'd been thinking for a while that mum could use a bigger place: between myself and Linda she now has five grandchildren and it's impossible for everyone to stay when we visit her, at Easter, or during the summer holidays.

Linda and I talk to mum about the idea of selling the house we grew up in and buying Whyte Avenue and, slightly to our surprise, she agrees. We complete in the summer of 2018.

As the final box was packed up at the old house, mum stood in the empty living room, quiet and thoughtful, running a hand along the mantelpiece that dad built in 1973, thinking about the forty-five years she'd spent in this place, about the life she made here, the family she raised, the two of them no longer here. She asked if we could leave her alone for a few minutes. Linda wandered out into the garden, with her own thoughts, and I headed upstairs. I climbed the metal stepladder to the attic.

It was still Gary's bedroom, almost exactly as he left it: the posters on the walls for club nights at the Pleasure Dome, at the Metro in Saltcoats. The grey-and-black 80s paint scheme. The old, dilapidated MFI wardrobe that his clothes hung in. I took the posters down and rolled them up in tubes, releasing flurries of dust, the motes hanging in the sunlight coming up through the trapdoor. I closed my eyes and sat there in the attic, cool even on this warm summer day, remembering, immersing myself in a random Saturday night from the early 90s. Everyone meeting up here for the pre-lash, on their way into town from their houses further out, on Hunter Drive, Kilwinning Road, Castlepark. The crack of cans of Red Stripe hissing open, spliffs being built on record sleeves and passed around, laughter and abuse fighting to be heard over Massive Attack or Gary Clail or Utah Saints coming from the wee portable record player in the corner. Dad banging on the metal ladder from down below, telling them to turn that bloody noise down. *'Sorry, Mr Niven!'* There's Keith and Larry and Peter Trodden and Tony and Paul Scott and wee Shades and they're wearing dungarees and Wallabees and –

Every single one of them dead and gone now.

Keith, Larry, Peter, Tony, Paul. And Gary. Heart attacks and cancer and overdose and suicide. All gone by their early fifties. The west coast of Scotland. The force of their laughter, their presence, still hangs around me up here. I say goodbye. I fold the metal ladder up, the three clanks as each section meets the other, and I push the carpeted trapdoor up with the stick and hear it snick shut for the very last time. Downstairs mum wipes a tear away, smiles bravely, and says, 'OK. Come on then.'

She begins another chapter of her life at the age of seventy-five, moving into Whyte Avenue in all its three-thousand-square-foot, four-bedroom, two-bathroom, two-reception-room, huge-gardened glory. Immediately, she loves living here. And it feels nice, to be able to do this. Tony Blundetto, buying Tony Soprano's house, no contract killing required. We throw a Christmas party at the end of the year, with an open bar and a whole roast lamb on a spit in the garden. Everyone comes, all the boys: Graham and Allan and Basil and Gordon and Rab and Peter and Andy Kerr and Andy Crone and Jim and all their wives and children, all of us in our early fifties now, all moving into late middle age, but their faces unchanged to me since we built a stage out of milk crates in my dad's garage nearly forty years ago. Across the living room, I watch mum talking to her eldest grandchild, Robin, now twenty-two.

She's holding a glass of champagne by the stem, her eyes bright, dancing with pleasure, as they always are at a party or treat of any kind. Three other grandchildren – Lila, Orlaith and Aoife, aged between six and ten – are running around being waitresses. A fifth, baby Alexandra, my youngest daughter, is asleep upstairs. Mum's parents, her husband, one of her sons, her two sisters, her brother, her brothers-in-law and

337

her aunts and uncles are all gone, but here she is, still eight stone dead and sipping Pol Roger in her new home. Living well is definitely the best revenge, although sometimes just living is enough. In the end it took five years and legal fees well into five figures until the Health Board understood that I would genuinely see them in court. As that date approached, in November 2015, they finally pled guilty to breaching health and safety legislation by failing to 'identify and implement adequate measures' to control the risk of 'patients with a mental health condition being left unattended in the accident and emergency department'. They were ordered to pay £67,000 in compensation and launch a 'root and branch review' of their procedures. Sheriff Livingston at Kilmarnock Sheriff Court found that 'Mr Niven lost his life in a way that was totally foreseeable' and said he would have fined the health board £100,000 had it not been for their guilty plea. The Chief Executive of Ayrshire and Arran Health Board John Burns said: 'I would like to take the opportunity to express our sincere condolences to the family of Gary Niven. We deeply regret the failures of the system that contributed to the sad death of Gary.' I got my legal costs back and we split the compensation largely between mum and Gary's son Dale, the boy finally getting some money from his father in death that he never got in life.

A Wee Roll and Butter

I rarely get any time back home without at least four children running around, and it's interesting to have the time and the quiet to observe mum's routines up close. Even though we bought her a big new smart TV for the main living room – pre-loaded with BBC iPlayer, Netflix and all the rest — she much prefers to watch television in the sun lounge, on her ancient flatscreen with just Freeview and a terrible, snowy picture. Much of this has to do with technology fear . . .

We finally got her an iPad the year before, as a way for her to see the grandkids more often, and she has gradually got to grips with FaceTime. Up to a point. Even after a year she still seems to have no sense of where the camera is, routinely filming her chest, stomach, chin or forehead, and most calls involve a few fraught minutes of 'no, higher, higher, look *into* the camera! The wee dot! Above the screen!' And God have mercy on your soul if you ever require her to film an object somewhere in the room — the wavering shots of ceiling and carpet, of blank wall and empty table-top. And then there's the way she interacts with the touchscreen itself: her finger jabbing at it in a crazy, pronounced, upward push, as though the screen is electrified, the jab turning into a finger point away from her, as though she is banishing an invisible demon to hell. It's like the exaggeratedly precise, firm way she pushes the buttons on an ATM or a card reader, the trembling forefinger rigidly extended, her free hand shielding her PIN digits as zealously as the swot guards their exam paper from the class cheat. And all the while a look of pain and alarm on her face, as though this time it will finally go wrong, as though typing in these four digits were the very maximum that could be asked of a human being.

Once again, I walk her through how to turn on the smart TV and get to Netflix, where she's keen to catch up with *The Crown*. 'Now you try,' I say, walking off to look at some emails. Within seconds, in the background, I can hear 'och!' and 'for God's sake!'

and 'aww, whit's it doing now?' I go back over and explain again. She gets it right this time, but I'm pretty certain the new TV will continue to gather dust when we're not around. When she does get the thing working mum's preferred viewing seems to involve alternating panel quiz shows with police procedurals. It crosses my mind that her ideal programme might well open with forensic officers in white paper suits talking to a world-weary cop by a bleak stretch of canal, before leading him into a crime scene tent . . . where Richard Osman raps his cards smartly on the desk before turning to camera. *Nine out of Ten Killings. The Pointless Murders.* Similarly, it is a quiz that brings her to the radio every morning, when she settles down to listen to Ken Bruce's *PopMaster* on Radio 2. Once again, despite the fact that there is a brand-new stereo with digital radio in the living room, mum prefers to listen to this on her cheap, ancient, badly tuned FM radio in the kitchen. At maximum volume. It is like hearing a wartime broadcast by Radio Free Europe on a crystal set during an air raid: the grating bursts of interference, the constant hiss and crump of static. But, like the dog who has lost its hind legs early in life, mum notices no significant diminishment in the quality of her existence. Indeed, she seems to feel there are certain goods you are allotted early in life and that to replace them unless they have become completely unusable would be incredibly wasteful, if not downright sinful. I once pointed out to her that her potato peeler was so bent and damaged it was painful to use. She sighed in a kind of what-can-you-do way, as though she were saying, 'I know this potato peeler isn't ideal, but it's the one I've been issued with' – the idea of spending, say, three quid on a new peeler being, presumably, a billionaire's dream.

Every morning as she listens to *PopMaster*, she has a pad and pen on her knee. At first, I think she is writing down her answers and find this odd as, to my knowledge, she has got maybe three questions right in two decades of listening to the show, routinely being stumped over brain-busters like 'name three hits by The Beatles' or 'John Travolta and Olivia Newton-John had a number one hit with "You're The One That I . . ."?' I go over and ask what she's writing down.

'Their scores,' she says, showing me the page.

'But, mum, they tell you what the score is.'

'Aye, well.'

'Do you think Ken might cheat them?'

'Och naw! It's just something I do.'

She goes off to put the kettle on and I flip back through her notepad. There are pages and pages of scorekeeping: four vertical strokes crossed with a diagonal mark, in the time-honoured way of keeping track of the days in prison. I am of a mind to mock this, but then I think of all the times I've listened to *PopMaster* and lost track of one of the contestants' scores and then not been listening when the round-up comes. Suddenly I am filled with huge affection for my mother doing this on a rainy Ayrshire morning, black coffee in one hand, biro in the other. It also occurs to me that if Ken Bruce ever finds himself at the centre of a historical cheating scandal, then right here, in Irvine, is a foolproof independent audit.

When it comes to food, for mum it is often the case of the simplest, fastest thing. A banana, a slice of toast or a cup of black instant coffee. One afternoon I come upon her buttering a roll in the kitchen. 'What are you making?' I ask.

'Just a wee roll and butter for ma lunch.'

This strikes me as spartan in the extreme. 'Would you like a ham salad roll?'

'Err . . .' She thinks about this strange, exotic offer for a moment. 'Aye, OK. That'd be nice.'

I slice a tomato, get some lettuce and ham out of the fridge, and add them to the roll with a pinch of salt and pepper. It takes roughly ninety seconds. 'Ooh, lovely,' mum coos, as I hand her the plate, as though Heston himself had just produced a side of beef that had spent twelve hours in the sous-vide.

I drive the seven minutes to the beach park and get out the car. The rain has stopped, the sun out now, but weak, as I cross the road and stand where it used to be.

They demolished the Magnum Centre three years ago, in 2017. A spokesman for North Ayrshire Council had said at the time: 'The demolition of the Magnum will allow the council to progress with its regeneration plans for the Irvine Harbour area and beyond, and form a component part of the ambitious proposals set out in the Ayrshire Growth Deal.' The huge site of the leisure centre is now just freshly planted grass, the earth still gouged and scarred here and there from the fearsome work of the heavy diggers. (Apparently, they removed tons of asbestos.) The site isn't even any use for social housing because of the warrens of old chemical mines deep below the surface. I look over to my right, to where the ice rink would have been and I can hear 'Mr Blue Sky', the air sharp and freezing in your lungs. I'm fifteen, clinging onto the side, teetering like a newborn colt in rented Purple Panthers as I watch Gary, just thirteen, just becoming Shades, zipping around in his sleek Bauer Hugger skates, his elbows pumping, his feet working economically, efficiently, just little squirts to the side. He comes speeding right up to me and clicks his twinned heels smartly to the side, stopping on a dime, sending a spray of freezing water and shaved ice all over me. The 'bastard!' is still forming on my lips when he's gone, laughing in a frosted cloud of breath.

I walk around the terrible blank expanse of grass, terrible in the way that, after an extraction, your tongue finds the jellied, salty hole where your tooth used to be. Outlived all usefulness. For years before the end, it had been a husk, a shell with the memories of former joys echoing inside it. It had just made it into its early forties and it was time to go, time for the wrecking ball. It reminds me of someone.

Using the old, elevated entrance bridge – still there, just hanging in space on the harbour side of the road – as a gauge, I work out where the sports hall would have been. And then, as best as I can, I work out where the stage would have been. And then the spot where the central microphone would have been. I stand there, roughly where Strummer would have stood, that night thirty-eight years ago. (And, oh Joe, I didn't realise until much, much later, but your brother killed himself too, didn't he? When you were just seventeen. There was no goodbye for you either.) No sea of drenched, ecstatic teenage faces to look out upon now. Just grass, the hillocks of the beach park in the distance, the Firth of Clyde beyond them. No matter. I close my eyes and I can hear that guitar ringing out, the chiming intro to 'Somebody Got Murdered' echoing off the chocolate-brown brick walls. I can hear the tom-toms pounding up as they come to join it, the bass beginning to throb, and then all of us are leaping into the air as one as the power chords and snare crash in together. Did Joe see any of us that night? Did he see our faces bathed in the lighting,

343

our eyes blown wide in wonder, mouths open, soaked to the skin, all of us as alive as it was possible to be? I look over and see three boys on bikes, about fifty yards away. They're fifteen, sixteen – the same age as the boys I have just been communing with – and they're looking my way.

Seeing what?

A mad old man, standing alone on a blasted patch of land, talking to himself. I fish for the keys as I head back towards the car, smiling.

This Pin – Two People

The odd things that set you off. Snow Patrol coming on Radio 2, in the car, years later. The song 'Run' – *'I'll be right beside you, dear.'* He used this word, repeatedly, to the 999 responder who answered the call. My daughter, with ice-cream on her hands, in front of Jeni's Ice Creams on Hillhurst in Los Angeles. As I wiped it off, telling her it might attract bees or wasps, I remember his hand, on the window of Mothercare on Kilmarnock High Street, on a hot day, covered in the strawberry Chewits he'd been eating. The wasp crawled down the glass and stung him. (Why were we in Mothercare? Mum must have been pregnant with Linda, making it the summer of 1973. He was almost five.) Three years after Gary died, during the tedium of a mortgage application process, I was forced into reviewing the previous three years' worth of accounts, something I would normally pay a great deal of money to avoid.

They included the returns for the tax year 2010–2011, encompassing the five months leading up to Gary's death. There were some alarmingly high figures underneath the (always elastic and ominous) heading 'travel and entertainment': a month-long Caribbean holiday in January 2010. Business-class flights to Los Angeles that summer. A week at the Chateau Marmont in Hollywood. Then there were the bigger, one-off purchases: the Mercedes estate, the car that had led to Gary getting the Saab, that had led to all that chaos and argument and tears. The garden office I had built. This was all during the same period that I chewed Gary out over the golf clubs business, that coded attempt to borrow four hundred quid, the same amount he later stole from mum. It occurred to me that almost any one of those things – the holidays, the car, the office – would probably have comfortably resolved my brother's debts. Thrashing now on hot, hostile sheets (maybe if you clamp a pillow between your legs, put one hand behind your back), I feel like Oskar Schindler in the third reel, as he stumbles around in front of his factory, the Deutsche Emailwarenfabrik, with his workforce, the saved, watching, sobbing, as he rants and raves – *'I could have done more . . . I threw away so much money . . . you have no idea . . . I didn't do enough . . . this car – why did I keep the car? Ten people right there. This pin – two people. At least one. I could have saved one more . . .'*

'Do you know anyone who'd buy my golf clubs?'

'Don't sell your golf clubs, Shades. How much do you need?'

That's how it should have gone. *'When there's room on my horse for two . . .'* But there wasn't. I just rode off, well-provisioned, and left him there, dying. I should have just put the cheque in the post without saying anything. For double – no, treble – the amount he needed. Why didn't I do that? Why did I have to mock him and belittle him and draw the words out of him? Eight hundred, a thousand, two thousand quid? Who would have cared now? What would it matter?

345

It might have bought him another few months. Maybe something would have happened. He might have retrained and got another job. Maybe his headaches would have got better. Maybe he'd have met a nice girl who'd have helped him get his life back on track. Maybe, maybe, maybe.

The Chernobyl of the soul.

I am impressed all over again by the half-life of suicide, by its power to go on and on and on. The book (the whodunnit? Or, rather, the whydunnit) with the last page torn out. The movie someone pulled the plug on fifteen minutes before the end. And then burned the negative. And shot everyone involved in the production. The director, the writer, the producer. The continuity person. The publicist. But, against all of this, there is the likely reality, the one that Linda and I can acknowledge only to each other, and then only quietly, when we're both in our cups: that things *wouldn't* have got better.

Indeed, would just have got worse as Gary got older, as his health and his temper and his finances deteriorated further and further. It would have been impossible to buy Whyte Avenue had he still been alive. There would have been his endless objections: *'Naw. We're no selling ma dad's house.'* He'd have fought so long, hard and bitterly against the scheme that mum would eventually have given in to him. Or he'd have insisted on Linda and I buying him out of his share of Livingstone Terrace. And then, a few years later, when he'd spent it all, he'd likely have wound up having to move into Whyte Avenue and live with mum anyway. Her and Eddie having dinner, or watching TV, while Gary's presence loomed around the house, angry and bitter, the air reeking of powerful weed, his voice rumbling from upstairs, on his mobile, putting together some fresh scheme. Mum, in her eighties, with the police at the door again. And then, far in the future, after mum died, there would be his inevitable attempt to claim sole ownership of the house. Because he'd lived there all those years. Because he'd done all this work to it. Because Gary wanted what he wanted. Then the tedious legal battle. Gary in his sixties, his seventies, like a mad old dog, crazier and more vicious. The drunken, abusive late-night phone calls. The fatwas issued against me and Linda for whatever slight, whatever perceived injustice. It is something we can only whisper to each other, brother to sister, the thing unsayable when it comes to the suicide of a difficult, troubled sibling, the one proudly clutching their fork as they stomp through a world of soup: *I'm glad he's dead.*

Oddly, there is some peace to be had from this stark, awful statement: to let them go, you must see them whole. And, after enough years have passed, you can reach, if not peace, then at least some kind of détente with The Questions. You come to understand that they will never stop and that the best you can do is to swim in them now and then. When they come, you let them flood you. They become less of a chorus of self-reproach and more of an affirmation that part of that person is still alive within you. You cannot bring them back, but you have not forgotten them. So, you stay with them a while, at your desk, in the car pulled over to the side of the road, with the song that reminded you of them playing on the radio.

I wake early the next morning, the tenth anniversary of Gary's death, and come downstairs for coffee just after 6.30am. It is already light outside, but grey and dark, the sky hanging low and heavy, swollen with unfallen rain, as it has been for much of the week. The last days of this lockdown summer have been a stark contrast to this time a decade ago, to the stunning weather that lasted for the entirety of the week of the coma, when I had played golf very early some mornings in conditions you rarely get up here, on the west coast of Scotland: ultra-still, not a breath of wind to stir the flagsticks or shimmer the long grass.

I come into the living room to see mum is already up. She is in her purple housecoat and is trying, with trembling hands and in the difficult way she sometimes has with inanimate objects, to light a small candle with a cigarette lighter. 'Och,' she says. 'For God's sake!'

I take it from her and light it. I get what is happening and ask, 'Do you always light a candle for Gary today, mum?'

'Aye, I try to, son,' she says. 'And on his birthday.'

Mum takes her candle over to the low shelf that runs the length of the living-room wall and sets it down next to a photograph of Gary, taken at night, on a balcony or terrace in a hot country (I think Mexico, but the only person who would know for sure would be the photographer – Leigh) nearly twenty years before. Shades is tanned – sunburnt in fact – and in his early thirties as he smiles for the camera, dressed in a clean white shirt and jeans, with a hand on his hip, his other arm leaning on the wall. It is the good times of the early 00s – after prison, before the disintegration. Beside it, inserted into the corner of the frame, is another photo of Gary, taken before Shades existed, when he was at primary school. He's in crew cut and sweater, eager, full of life and cheek. Another photograph nearby, of me and Gary, aged six and four, down the moors, at Marymass. My arm around him, protectively. *Because you were meant to protect him.* 'There you are, son,' mum says. 'Ah hope you're at

348

peace now.' She sighs, looking at the photographs, the glass of the frames rippling orange-yellow in the candlelight, the weak dawn coming through the blinds, the smirr drizzling on the windowpanes. Dreich. 'Ah hope your demons are all behind you,' she says.

Mum touches the frame gently, remembering . . . what? The good times? The bad times? The beginning? The end? *That honking, rasping snoring.*

I try to imagine it, the thing you dread the most from the moment you hear their first cries, the moment you hear the words 'It's a boy!' or 'It's a girl!'

The death of the child.

Robin, Lila, Alexandra or Morty, breathing their last as the monitors tick their way down to nothing. Putting a hand on the fevered brow as the life leaves them. Watching them go forever, having never recovered consciousness, without having heard you say the things you so badly needed them to hear one last time.

I love you.

I love you so much.

You were my beautiful wee boy.

No. You shake your head and blow your cheeks out. Your bum fizzing as you chase it away. Just a nightmare. Not reality, not memory. Not what mum is dealing with right now, here on the living-room carpet. 'I just . . .' she'd said the night before as we sat finishing our wine. 'If he'd just opened his eyes for a minute. Just for a minute.' Replaying that non-minute every day for the rest of your life. I get up quietly from the sofa, cross the room, and put my arms around her, folding her into me. She's so small now, tiny and fragile. I say the words she said to us in childhood, countless times.

'It's OK,' I whisper. 'Don't cry. It'll be all right . . .'

We stay like that for a while, me holding her, pressed against her back, with my eyes closed, smelling her hair. *Harry by the Sea*, in the armchair by the window at Martin Avenue, savouring the mum smell I have known for as long as I have known consciousness. Gary watches us, smiling, the candlelight flickering across his face, on the terrace in some hot country I can't quite be sure of. He watches us, mum and I, locked in embrace. *If we could have been there with you, that night, would it have made a difference?*

GARY

Tuesday, 31 August 2010 – 1.05am

He feels it coming, worming its way up towards him through the dream-murk. It wakes him as it always does, around ninety minutes after he's fallen asleep, alone in the middle of a double bed, in the middle of the night, in the middle of his life. The circadian rhythm, that doctor said, the ophthalmic nerve. He feels it first as a presence lurking somewhere behind his right eye, as though something is feeling its way out from the middle of his brain, searching for escape. He steels himself, getting ready. Ah fuck, man, fuck sake. He starts grinding his knuckles into the ocular cavity. Helps. It's like it's in there, like a splinter. Christ, getting worse. Just lie here a minute. He's sweating lightly in the cold bedroom, his right eyelid fluttering as the pain finally crackles away to nothing.

He tries to get back to sleep, but his own voice won't leave him alone: *Whit are you gaunnae dae, Shades?* Money's gone. She's no noticed yet, been a week. She's bound tae soon, ya daft bastard. Whit are ye gaunnae say to her? *'Naw, hen. No me. Honest, maw. Somebody must have broke in.'* Jist tell her the truth – *'Ah'm sorry. Ah'll huv it back tae ye in a couple o' weeks.'* Cannae sleep noo. Get up – make a wee roll-up? Nae hash left. Hud a hale cupboard full o' grass. Court date coming soon fur that. Second offence. Just weed, man. Still, get the wrang

353

judge . . . No way, man. Imagine it? Maw going through aw that again? Feels like you're going mad.

He gets up, his feet finding the slippers beside the bed. He is already fully clothed. Has been sleeping like this for a while now. Thanks to the headaches, he rarely gets more than an hour or two at a stretch anyway. *Freezing in here.* Need tae top the key up. Downstairs, in the kitchen, he automatically goes to put the kettle on. Then remembers. Gets a glass of water at the kitchen sink instead. Nae milk and sugar even if there was electricity. Drinking the water in the darkness of the kitchen, he looks through to the living room – there it was, on the dining table: more and more o' the broon envelopes. Didnae even open them now. Whit wiz the point? Cannae get blood oot a stane. Forty-two years oan the planet and this is it, Shadesy boy, aw ye've goat tae show – some jeans and taps and an Xboax. Naw, there wiz something else. There wiz Dale. *Aye, and maybe the rest – a few weans aboot this toon wi' your face.* Naw – don't think aboot that either. The garage. Come oan. Just have a look at it.

Stepping into the breeze-blocked space. Cold. Even colder than the house. His torchbeam lights it up – the metal stepladder standing in the middle, where the car he never had would be. Above it, dangling from the beam, the noose of thin, blue nylon clothesline. Three steps up and he takes it in his right hand and slips it over his head. He leans forward, testing his weight on it, feeling the pressure around his throat, the rough, prickly nylon biting into his flesh. They say ye piss yersel. Maybe get a hard-oan an aw. Cheap thrill. Aye – no sae cheap, but. Dae it oot here, leave the note in the hoose: *'Maw, don't go in the garage. Just call the police. Gary x.'* Step aff. Aw be over in a few minutes. Naw. Ah don't want tae. *Come oan, ya fanny – just dae it.* Naw.

354

Back into the house. He goes through to the living room, lights the candles on the coffee table, and gets his baccy tin. The wee sticker in the middle, the words 'fuck off' in tiny letters in a circle. Red-eyed, exhausted, he makes the roll-up, enough left for maybe two mair. Then how long till the giro? Then the voice is saying – *the kit's right there oan the coffee table, wee boy.* He sits down on the edge of the sofa and picks up one of the three Stanley knives. He starts pressing the point into the inside of his forearm. Even though it's quite blunt, it's enough to draw blood – a line appearing, dark as that Bucky in the fridge. Could ye – just push down hard. *Shut your eyes and do it.* They say you should do it in a warm bath. Like yer man in *The Godfather. Warm bath?* Nae chance o' that. Scottish Power cunts. But the mess, man. Maw might come up. Still goat a key. Just dae it, slide the knife across and – *fuck sake, Shades. How did it get tae this?* He picks up his mobile – just a watch now, nae credit – and sees it's nearly four o'clock in the morning. Still pitch-black outside. The living-room windows face the back garden. The sun comes up around five, at the front, through the kitchen window. Darkest hour an aw that. Just get through this fucking night. And then . . . and then what?

Mair envelopes.

Mair headaches.

Court dates.

Son that disnae know ye fae Adam.

'For ma retirement.'

Whit did dad say? 'Ye'll end up a bum, Gary. A bloody bum.' Battered ye under the living-room table. Ye telt him tae go fuck himself, so ye did. Was gaunnae hook him. But ye wurnae far wrang, auld yin –

gaunnae end up doon Cunny House right enough, wi' the rest o' the dross. Just press it down, here. Push it across . . . over they big veins. *Oh, help me, da. Maw. Ah want away fae here. Ah want tae go home.* Before he really knows what he's doing he puts the Stanley knife down on the coffee table, picks up his mobile, and dials the number, the same three digits in a row, pressed down with the thumb of the right hand. The one number you don't need any credit for.

'Police, Fire, Ambulance – which service do you require?'

'Err, aye, ambulance, please.'

A moment, and then a woman comes on the line. She's middle-aged. Nice-sounding. 'Hello, Ambulance Service, what's the address of the emergency?'

'Ah, it's five Birkscairn Place, Bourtreehill, Irvine.'

'Five which place?'

'Bourtreehill, five Birkscairn Place, Bourtreehill.'

'Is that a main door or a flat?'

'It's a main door, please.'

'And what's the telephone number you're calling from?'

'Oh, it's oh-treble seven-eight-seven-five . . .'

'Mmm . . .'

'. . . four-nine-seven-two.'

'Thank you, and just confirm the address again for me?'

Fuck sake. 'It's five Birkscairn Place, Bourtreehill.'

'And what's the problem there?'

'What's that?'

'What's the problem there?'

'What's the property near?'

'No, what's the problem? Why do you need an ambulance?'

356

'Eh, Ah . . . Ah've been suffering fae depression, dear, because Ah lost my job a long time ago.'

'Mmm.'

'Ah cannae find work, eh?'

'Mmm.'

'Ah've just tried tae slash my wrists and hang maself.'

'So, you're going to hang yourself? How old are you?'

'Forty-one, dear.' *(He is forty-two. Vanity? Confusion?)*

'I'm just going to ask you a few quick questions, I'm not delaying any help for you. One of my colleagues is arranging the help while I'm speaking to you. Are you feeling violent towards anyone?'

'I'm what?'

'Are you feeling violent towards anyone?'

'No, no.'

'No?'

'Just myself, dear.'

'Are there any weapons there?'

'Aye.'

'What weapons do you have?'

'Aye, I've got three Stanley knives in front of me.'

'Three Stanley knives.' *(At this point, following procedure, the responder alerts the police, who will accompany the ambulance crew.)* 'And whereabouts in the house are you?'

'Eh, in the living room.'

'Living room.'

'Aye. Ah was out my garage trying tae hang maself and couldnae dae it and I came back in and Ah took some Stanley knives and Ah've just been trying tae cut my throat. Ma . . . ma wrists.'

357

'OK, I'm organising the help for you now. Stay on the line and I'll tell you exactly what to do next.'

'OK.'

'Help has been arranged for you. Don't have anything to eat or drink. It might make you sick or cause problems for the doctor. Just rest in the most comfortable position for you. Now, I'm going to give you some instructions before I let you go. If you can, put away any family pets, gather any medication you're on, unlock the door, and if anything changes, you call us back immediately for further instructions. What's your name?'

'It's Gary. Gary Niven.'

'Gary Niven. That's fine, Gary. We've got all the help arranged for you, OK?'

'Right.'

'Thanks, bye-bye now.'

'Right, bye, dear. Thanks.' *(He calls her 'dear' four times, an anachronism also used by mum.)*

'You're welcome.'

She hangs up.

Through those windows, a couple of miles northwest of here, mum, sleeping. Or not. Like you these days. Only gets a couple of hours a night if she's lucky. *Aye – and how many o' those sleepless nights huv you caused? Her lying there, crying herself tae sleep, thinking about ye going tae yer bed in the Bar-L? Thinking about . . .*

A few minutes pass, and then a soft blue light is falling across the dining table, gently illuminating the drift of hell-mail. It fades away and comes back. Fades and comes back.

He gets up and walks to the doorway to see the ambulance parked in front of the house, its strobing lights filling the kitchen, like being

358

inside a blue water pistol. Mind the smell o' a water pistol when ye were wee? When ye put yer nose to the hole when ye were filling it up? Smelt aw brand new and – haud on – the polis here an aw? Fuck sake – how come? After the other week, the raid, the neighbours . . . he walks towards the front door just as the knocking starts. Opens it.

'Mr Niven? Gary?' the first guy says. 'Can we come in?'

'Aye, aye, pal.'

Four o' them there. Two ambulance guys and two polis. Whit are the polis daeing here? As though reading what he's thinking, the big polis says, 'Do you have weapons in the house, Gary? Knives?' Woman oan the phone must have said. Fuck, upstairs, in the drawer. The–

'Naw. Well, aye, but no really . . .'

They follow you through to the living room, to the glow of the candles. 'Do you mind if we turn the lights on, Gary?' one of them asks.

'Naw, pal, Ah wouldnae mind, but Ah've nae electricity. Nae money fur the meter. The wee key, ken?'

'OK, not a problem.'

They're turning on their torches, looking around. The police see your blunt, feeble Stanley knives are all they have to worry about. They pick them up and retreat down the hall, leaving the ambulance crew to their work. Big guys, green uniforms, padded, loads of kit hanging aff them. 'We'd better look at that arm then, eh?'

'Aye, aye,' you say, as if noticing it for the first time.

'Do you want to tell us what happened tonight, Gary?' the one examining your arm says.

'Jist, eh, aye, like Ah said tae the wummin oan the phone, Ah've no been able tae find any work, ken? Ah'm behind oan aw ma bills

359

and . . . there wiz a pal o' mine died no long ago, motorbike crash. Ma heid's been bad. Ah get these cluster headaches and they've been bad this past three, four days. No slept much. Disnae seem tae be much point going on . . .' The guy's dabbing cream, antiseptic, oan there. Stings. Starting to bandage it. Isnae even bleeding much now. Getting these boys oot here fur this? 'Ah set up a noose oot there in ma garage, ken?' he says, hoping to make it sound like a more worthwhile trip.

'Can I just look into your eyes, please?'

'Aye.' He gets the wee light out and shines it in there. The other wan's radio is crackling and he steps out into the hall to answer it. 'Have you been drinking tonight, Gary?'

'Naw, naw. It's bad fur ma headaches. Ah've hud a half-bottle o' Bucky sitting in the fridge fur ages so Ah huv. Cannae face it.'

'Have you taken anything else? Drugs?'

'Naw. Aye, sometimes a wee bit o' puff, ken? But no fur a while. No hud the money.'

He's finished examining you, bandaging you. It really hasn't taken very long. The other guy comes back into the room. It feels like you need to say more. 'Ah'm jist . . . Ah'm feart Ah'm gaunnae dae something tae maself. Something daft, ken?'

I just want someone to come and take me away.

They look at each other. Come to a decision.

'OK, Gary, we're going to take you to hospital, to Crosshouse, to see a doctor. Can you walk?'

'Aye, aye.'

The back of the ambulance, tightly packed technology. One of them sits across from you as you come along snaking Birkscairn Way and then turn left on Towerlands Road, heading east, towards Springside. You can see up ahead that the sun is starting to rise now. Another warm day. Maybe you'll get a bed. Three hot meals. Just be like . . . a wee holiday. A flicker through his skull again, like that nerve just got pulled tight. Aw fuck. Here we go. He covers his face, fingertips digging into his right temple, and sits forward, rocking, the first moans coming out.

'Gary, are you OK?' the guy says.

'Naw, wan o' ma headaches. Ahh, fuck . . . can . . . can I huv some o' that oxygen? Ah've got a prescription fur it. Honest.'

The guy fiddles with a tank and then hands him the mask. He starts breathing deeply, sucking it right in, the way the doctor told him to, at the hospital in London that time.

But this attack doesn't last long and soon he's looking up with watering eyes to see they are pulling into the car park – Crosshouse appearing up ahead. He follows the paramedics into A&E and takes a seat in a corridor while they talk with a nurse. *('Half-hearted suicide attempt,' one of the paramedics will say to her.)* 'OK, Gary,' one of them says. 'We'll leave you with these guys. Hope you feel better soon.'

'Aye, thanks, boys. Sorry, ken? Ah'm sorry for all the bother.' He wonders vaguely what this trip will have cost. Thousands tae call oot an ambulance he's heard.

'Not at all.' They head back out.

The nurse sits down beside him and reads through the notes the ambulance guys have given her. 'Just let me look at those cuts again, Gary.'

As she unwinds the dressing, she talks to him, asking him what happened tonight, and he finds himself going through it all for the third time: nae work, nae money, debts, headaches, his pal's motorbike crash. The noose in the garage. The Stanley knives. She bandages his arm back up and takes him through to a small room, a white cubicle, hot, strip lights blaring, his skull immediately giving a forbidding pulse. 'OK. If you take a seat in here, Gary, a doctor will be along to see you as soon as they can.'

'Aye, Ah've been having bad headaches the night, but. Can Ah get some oxygen? Just in case?'

'That'd need to be prescribed by the doctor.'

'They gave it tae us in the ambulance!'

'You'll need to wait to see the doctor.'

Fuck sake. This auld boot. 'Ah, fuck – aye, awright.'

He sits down and she walks away, leaving the door open as she goes to talk to a couple of other nurses over there, sitting at their wee station. Oh, man, so tired. The room is like a prism. White walls. Fluorescent tubes. He feels it coming again, like a dial getting turned up and up. Aww tae fuck – naw, naw, naw. That dagger, sliding into the eyeball from behind. Oh Jesus Christ, this isnae real. He gets up and staggers through the open door, towards the two nurses. 'Ah need oxygen! Please. Fur ma heid!'

'The doctor will see you soon,' one of them says.

'F–' He wants to kick off, to say, 'AH'M IN AGONY HERE! HOW COME THEY GIED IT TAE US IN THE AMBULANCE FUR FUCK SAKE!'

But he sees the signs all over the place – *'Abuse will not be tolerated.'* Might call the polis. He storms back into the cubicle, the headache ratcheting up even more. He tries sitting on the floor. Banging his head on the wall. Fucking cows. Jist oxygen. (In the full Ayrshire: *'oaks-ay-gin'*.)

Whit harm can it do? He looks up through the open doorway and sees the two nurses are gone, both away to deal with something.

Nae oxygen?

Sit doon and shut up?

Half-hearted?

Ah'll show yese half-hearted.

He looks around the room: a wee step stool sitting there. In a moment it assumes sentience. Full lethality.

An executioner.

Aye, Shades. Ah dare ye. Ah fucken double dare ye, wee man.

You cross the room – three steps – and gently close the door. No one's watching. You're alone in here. *You've been alone for so long now.*

You get your sweater off – *armies uppa sky!* – the grey skinny-rib Ralph Lauren Polo a relic of happier times, when you were a player, and quickly tie the arms into a kind of loop, a noose. There's another door, at the back. Just opens onto another wee room. It's empty. You open the door and hook the loop end around that. Close the door, jamming it in there. Up on the stool. The other end around your neck. *Jist make it stop for a minute.* You step off the stool and kick it away. Your first feeling is surprise. Surprise that the sweater doesn't rip, that it's really holding you, your feet magically pedalling just inches off the linoleum floor. You can't breathe. You can't get your feet on the floor. Can't reach up to unhook yourself. Can't work your fingers into the woollen noose around your neck. And all of this from your sweater on a door! Imagine what that clothesline out in your garage would have done. You start to struggle, pedalling frantically in mid-air. You're the Roadrunner. Mind that? Saturday mornings on the wee portable telly. You've charged right off that cliff edge. *Beep! Beep!* Panic kicks in now as you start scrabbling at that noose. But it's pulled much, much too tight. And now that physics has done its work – your ten stones dropping a foot through the air with a ligature around your neck, many terrible kilos of pressure being applied to your fragile airway – it's biology's turn to step forward, with its mad parade of Latin names . . .

Hypoxia. You are simply not getting enough oxygen. Your brain (o selfish organ!) is trying to conserve what little there is for itself, and for that other king: your heart, which is pumping crazy-fast as it tries to increase the output of oxygenated blood. The conservation effort going on for these two principalities means that less and less blood is going to the provinces, to the peripheral tissue, which is why you are already starting to turn blue. Soon enough the princes – your kidneys and liver – are also beginning to struggle.

Pulmonary oedema. Your blood pressure is going through the roof, increasing the workload on your poor lungs. Tattered from nearly thirty years of Kensitas Club, from decades of scorching hashish and leafy green weed, they're literally sweating from exertion, like an out-of-shape jogger. Fluid is pouring down their walls, gradually filling them up, further reducing their capacity, their ability to manufacture fresh oxygen. All of this is worsening an already very bad situation and quickly leading you towards . . .

Cerebral ischemia. There just isn't enough blood flowing to your brain to meet metabolic demand. This is causing a cerebral infarction. You feel like a tube of toothpaste someone is trying to get the last drop out of, everything being forced to the top with fat thumbs, but with the cap still tightly on. It's like your fucking head is going to explode.

Your thoughts are ranging madly, popping all over the place. Why? Because you are now having a massive stroke. Vast areas of your brain are beginning to be wiped out, like brushfire sweeping through dry heather. Your struggling slows and it takes less than a minute for you to begin to lose consciousness. The real world is zipping away from you like a reverse zoom – Chief Brody on the beach – as everything becomes internal. Suddenly there are fireworks. Galaxies and spangled constellations are unfolding across the blackness behind your eyelids. You are going to Ultra! *Under the covers. Rub your knuckles into your eyes. It's like going into space!* The universe comes rushing towards you – purple starbursts, blue shimmers, exploding galaxies. You chase after them, bounding down the rabbit hole. You're all laughing, in the car, the old navy Cortina, going on holiday. Mum would make you a surprise box, give it to you once you were on the road: comics and sweeties and a wee carton of juice. The man's hand, lifting the model planes out that window, then she came out and gave them to us. Spooning the rusks towards you – *'here comes an aeroplane!'* – picking you up in the middle of the night, nursing you over her shoulder as she looked out that window onto the back courtyard at Martin Avenue. Her hand, patting your back, soft and rhythmic. *There, there, Gary, son. Shh now.* She was twenty-five. *Ah'm sorry, maw. Sorry aboot yer money. It's better this way, hen, yer better aff. Ah jist couldnae handle it aw any mair.* Linda. *Linda.* Fuck. *Aww, hen, wee girl, Ah'm sorry, Ah'm sorry so Ah um. Ma ain wee sister. Ah shouldnae have done aw that stuff. Whit kind o brother wiz Ah tae ye?* And you find you can say all this now – nothing matters. You feel free. The terrible present and the awful future are receding and all you have are these random bits of the past, all thrown together, jumbled nonsense, like when you're falling asleep, or like on glue – *Happy Birthday, Danny!* – all coming at you and then fast disappearing as frames get caught in the projector, flaring up into blue and red bubbles, then blowing out, whiteout, gone forever.

But not forever, because I'm here, remembering them for you.

You're in the woods, in your tent, the smell of the beans over the fire, the moon up there, low above the trees. The moon low that other night, years later, as you walked back tae yer cell, just a big pewter disc over the prison, the bottom of its bright ring fringed jaggy black by the barbed wire. Wee Dale, born when ye were in there. Last time ye saw him, going doon the path. Bye, son. Bye, daddy, bye-bye. *Aww, wee man. Ah'm sorry. Ah wiz always thinking aboot ye.* Now you're dancing, up the Pleasure Dome, the smoke and the strobes and the music and the green lasers raking your face, aw loved up wi' aw yer pals; Larry and Peter and Tony and Paul and Dykes and Budgie and Vouchers and everyone. Maw and Bell and Emily dancing – *yessirI-canboogie* – and you all up in the wee den at Whyte Avenue with the Tennent's and the McEwan's. *The SHADES from a pencil peer!* Then you can feel rubber between your thighs. You're wearing shorts. You're on Mungo! You're hurtling downhill on Martin Avenue, blinded by the summer sunshine, the burnt toffee of creosote and the new carpet smell of cut grass and the rubber dog smelling like wet biscuits, smelling like 1971, as you go faster and faster, the baked concrete unspooling beneath you, your feet held up above the wheels, the houses flashing past on either side, other weans cheering you on, someone – mum? John? – shouting for you to slow down, to stop. But you'll never do that. Shadesy-boy? Gary Niven? Stop? Hit the brakes? Nae chance, wee sacks. *Wheeeeeee!* And then you're tipping over, falling, falling forwards, still gripping the handles, nothing to stop you, the crystalline

366

chips in the black tarmacadam glittering like diamonds as the ground rushes up to meet your nose, your milk teeth.

A nurse is screaming in the doorway now, but it's nothing to you, no more than someone coughing three rooms away.

You find you can remember *everything*. You're looking up at the moon, through a window, you're safe and warm, all bundled up, someone's holding you, and John's there, right next to you. *There's men walking around up there.* Just as you remember these words, a face is coming out of the freezing blackness up ahead, out of whatever fresh universe you're heading into now. Grey-white hair, like smoke, the seamy forehead, the big, broad nose, the pores getting bigger as the face comes closer, like screw holes, then plugholes, then manholes. God. It's not God. It's . . . it's *him*. You thought he'd be angry, the bottom teeth bared, the jaw taut and jutting. But he's not. He . . . he's *smiling*, full of joy. Pals again. Like when you were wee, out in the back garden with the football. He has no body now, no limbs, and neither do you, but even so, you can feel him reaching out, feel yourself being folded into his arms. He is huge and you are tiny as his smells envelop you – Swarfega and Embassy Regal and Old Spice and the Grouse that was Famous. And finally, after all these years, after all the drink and the ecstasy and the speed and the coke and the Valium and the antidepressants and the jellies and the smack and the doctors and psychiatrists and the punched walls and slammed doors it's here, the only thing that would ever have helped anyway. You're both getting to say it all, now, at the end, getting the words out in voices stained by tears . . .

'Ah'm sorry. Ah made a mess of everything, so Ah did. Ah should huv listened tae ye. Ah should huv stuck in at the school, Ah should huv tried harder . . . Ah . . . I love you, daddy.'

'Shh, wee man. It's ma fault. Ah shouldnae huv lost ma temper wi' ye aw they times. Ah shouldnae huv hit ye. It's OK. It'll be all right. Don't cry. I love you too, son.'

And it is blissful, as the word 'son' falls upon you like absolution, warm and soft. You can feel it all leaving you, the guilt and the rage and the sadness and the pain. Like when the headaches lift. Dad is carrying you, a baby in his arms again, like Superman as he drives fearlessly into the darkness ahead, past the red giants and yellow dwarfs and black holes that are coming zooming faster and faster towards you across the vastness of space, carrying you towards that place where nothing matters any more, where everything will finally be all right.

The event horizon.

And then you're slipping over it.

You're both gone.

Vanishing into something like love.

Resources

International suicide prevention helplines can be found at befrienders.org. In the UK and Ireland, Samaritans can be contacted on 116 123 or email jo@samaritans.org or jo@samaritans.ie. Other charities include Mind: mind.org.uk and CALM: thecalmzone.net. In the US, the National Suicide Prevention Lifeline is at 800-273-8255 or chat for support. You can also text HOME to 741741 to connect with a crisis text line counselor. In Australia, the crisis support service Lifeline is 13 11 14.